Why Can't I Lose Weight?

by

Lorrie Medford, C.N.

LDN Publishing
P.O. Box 54007
Tulsa, Oklahoma 74155

Unless otherwise indicated, all Scripture quotations are taken from the *King James Version* of the Bible.

Medford, Lorrie, 1949
        Why Can't I Lose Weight?
    Lorrie Medford
    Includes bibliographical references
    International Standard Book Number: 0-9676419-0-X
    1.Weight loss. 2. Nutrition. 3. Diet. 4. Health. 5. Reducing Diets.
    6. Reducing—Religious Aspects—Christianity

The information presented in this book is intended as an informative resource guide to help you make informed decisions. It is not meant to replace the advice of a physician or to serve as a guide to self-treatment. Always seek competent medical help for any health condition or if there is any question about the information presented. Every effort has been made to provide accurate information. The author assumes no responsibility for any outcome of applying this information in this book by an individual or with a licensed health care professional.

NOTE: This program is designed for healthy adults. If you have special health needs such as chronic disease, diabetes, heart conditions, pregnancy or are a lactating woman, or have a medical condition that requires medical attention, consult your health care provider for assistance and advice before beginning this program.

Printed in the United States of America

10 9 8 7 6 5 4 3 2 1 First U.S. Edition

(For ordering information, refer to the back pages of this book.)

Dedication

This book is dedicated to my family—my identical twin sister, Jackie Johnson—my big sis, Rabia Fournier, and my mother, Donna Van Every, who taught me the value of persistence, goals, and an up-to-date library card. Thanks for your precious love and encouragement.

I wrote this book for my clients! So often I wish I had this book in my office during a counseling session so we could turn to a page to get clearer understanding about something. I pray this book is a blessing to you on your journey to health and weight loss!

Contents

PART SIX: WHAT DO HORMONES HAVE TO DO WITH WEIGHT LOSS?

PART SEVEN: WHAT SHOULD I EAT?

PART EIGHT: GO FOR IT!

Foreword

I am honored to have Lorrie Medford as an active member of our church. Her lifestyle and consistent, overcoming attitude is a great example to other believers, and her sincere love for people is contagious.

This book has been one of the most complete and practical books on nutrition I have ever seen. It's obvious it has been written from thousands of hours of research and experience.

Even if in the past you have tried diets and weight loss programs that have caused you to become discouraged and give up, this book will be different. You will be encouraged and not feel condemned with these simple keys that are livable and relevant. God has a vibrant, rich life ahead for you.

If we are going to accomplish the vision and destiny He has for us, a healthy body, clear mind and an abundance of physical energy is essential. This book is really life changing.

—PASTOR EASTMAN CURTIS
DESTINY CHURCH
TULSA, OKLAHOMA

Acknowledgments

My heartfelt thanks and gratitude go to:

My family: Rabia Fournier, Jackie and Bob Johnson, and my mother, Donna Van Every, and the Van Every Family—my aunts, uncles, and cousins in Buffalo, New York.

All of my clients for believing in the gift in me and allowing me to serve you.

Special thanks to the people who took my weight loss classes throughout the last ten years at any of these locations: Tulsa Junior College, Akins Natural Foods Market, Grace Fellowship, Planet Fitness, and Life Design Nutrition.

Much gratitude to the many authors, researchers and nutritionists whose books I have studied throughout the years. Thank you for allowing me to quote you.

Special thanks to Donald Warren, D.D.S., for your thoughtful reading of my entire manuscript. Also many thanks to nutritionist Dr. Lindsey Duncan, scientist Brian Scott Peskin, and author Cheryl Townsley. Thanks you for willingness to find time to read my manuscript! Your comments and feedback helped to make this book more readable and valuable.

Walter Scott and Glenn Kikel from Standard Process Labs. Thanks for your continual support, encouragement and help with continuing education on nutrition.

Susie Hooke for your generous assistance with the shopping chapter.

Many thanks to Brandon Sensintaffar for your wonderfully creative work on the cover.

Thank you so very much, Lisa Simpson, for the hours you spent so willingly proofreading. You are a great encourager!

My pastors, Eastman and Angel Curtis from Destiny Church in Tulsa, Oklahoma. I am grateful for the love and faith you show us as you walk out *your* destiny. Your constant encouragement is a continual blessing.

Thank you for believing in me and the gift in me.

Most of all, I thank the Living God, without Whom I am nothing, and I can do nothing.

About the Author

Lorrie Medford has a B.A. in Communications and is a licensed Certified Nutritionist from The American Health Science University. She also holds a certification as a personal trainer from ISSA (International Sports Science Association).

A health researcher and journalist, Lorrie has studied nutrition, whole-foods cooking, herbs, health, fitness, and motivation for more than twenty years. Lorrie taught her weight loss class for more than nine years, and has taught natural foods cooking classes for three years.

She shares her knowledge not only in this book, but in her seminars, and through her nutritional consultation practice, Life Design Nutrition in Tulsa, Oklahoma.

Lorrie is uniquely qualified to write about health and fitness. She knows what it's like to be a cranky calorie counter obsessed with foods, dieting, and striving to be thin. After struggling with her weight for many years, Lorrie lost thirty-plus pounds and has kept the weight off for more than fourteen years by following the ideas presented in this book. She has also written a motivational weight loss book, *Why Can't I Stay Motivated?* and *Why Can't I Lose Weight Cookbook?*

Lorrie has a rich history of community involvement teaching nutrition and is a sought-after speaker for civic groups, churches and wellness organizations.

Know the truth and the truth shall set you free.

John 8:32, NLT

We Can All Win the "No-Belly" Prize!

As a Certified Nutritionist, I am amazed that even though hundreds of books on diet, fitness, and compulsive behaviors regularly flood the marketplace, Americans are not downsizing!

Millions of Americans are still overweight, and those who do lose weight regain it within a short time. Why are we still losing the war on fat?

I've Been There!

I know what it's like to be obsessed with foods, dieting and being thin. I know what it's like to try program after program looking for the magic solution to weight loss. Like thousands of others, I was an unsuccessful, cranky calorie counter. I know how frustrating it was when the buttons came off my favorite jeans—or, when I would go on a diet and the only thing I really lost was my patience!

No Longer Obsessed

Twenty years ago I started reading books on health, nutrition, and diet, and at fifty, I'm in better shape and healthier than I was as a teenager. I've lost more than thirty pounds and have kept the weight off for fourteen years. Even more importantly, I've lost my cravings for junk food, my overeating patterns, and my obsession with food. I no longer want to live my life wishing I had someone else's hips and thighs!

Get Healthy First

I am confident that you can lose weight, too. After winning the battle over weight myself, and helping people over the past ten years, I believe that for many people, *weight loss is primarily a health issue.* Emotional or spiritual counseling is valuable, and I often recommend this to my clients. But I have been surprised at how many of my clients' food cravings fell away when we dealt with conditions like poor digestion, balancing blood sugar levels and food allergies.

Design Your Life

To lose weight permanently requires two things: (1) Discover what's been hindering your weight loss, and (2) make it a lifestyle this time.

A healthy diet, along with healthy eating patterns, needs to become a lifestyle—a way of life. I named my nutritional counseling business Life Design Nutrition because unless we make changes that we are going to do for the rest of our lives, they won't last—changes like how you think about food, shopping, preparing meals, and eating.

What's the Problem?

In this book, I share what I have found to be physical causes of obesity and tell you how to deal with them. You'll learn how to:

1. Eliminate poor digestion
2. Banish constipation
3. Improve your fat-burning ability
4. Energize your body and eliminate fatigue
5. Conquer food cravings
6. Balance your hormones

More Than "Just Say No"

I'm convinced that it's not just a matter of eating smaller portions, having willpower, or saying "no," although these actions help. For many people, losing weight may be more of a health problem than a self-discipline problem. There are several physical imbalances that cause people to crave sugars.

Handle the Imbalances

My balanced plan helps people eat well, eliminates cravings, and produces more energy almost immediately. We'll explore a way of eating that encourages fat metabolism, and I'll give you menu-planning ideas, recipes, and a shopping list.

15

My plan is easy-to-follow, simple, effective, and livable! My approach is based on foods that are satisfying. The exciting thing is that my weight-loss clients not only lost weight safely, naturally, and kept it off, but they reaped many other benefits: better digestion, lowered triglyceride and cholesterol levels, healthier blood-sugar levels, and increased energy. The foods that burn body fat often have the potential to help protect you from cancer, diabetes, and other diseases.

You Can Do It!

A vital aspect of weight loss is motivation. Part of the reason I was able to lose the weight was because I was motivated. I'm not perfect. I fudge from time to time. But I still lost weight and have kept it off for many years. Throughout this book, I have written motivational statements to get you started and encourage you along the way. A summary of these motivational statements is in Appendix A.

I know I'll never have a weight problem again as long as I continue to follow the principles presented in the following pages. And I believe you can succeed, too.

Take Small Steps

Broken into eight parts, this book presents a step-by-step plan. It shows you what to do, why to do it, and how to do it. I recommend you start with Parts One and Two. If you don't want to read the entire book, then go to Part Eight. Otherwise, read the book in order.

Part One is your basis for understanding why we struggle with weight loss. You'll learn why all fad diets are doomed to fail.

Part Two will show you the top three causes for overweight and what you can do about them.

Part Three presents the facts about thermogenic products and the value of supporting your thyroid gland.

Part Four gives the most common reasons for fatigue, including allergies, low blood sugar, and Candida Albicans.

Part Five helps you to beat many food cravings.

Part Six helps you balance your hormones, another hidden cause of overweight.

Part Seven tells you how and why to eliminate foods that are causing you to store fat.

Part Eight gives my basic principles for healthy eating, and a six-week eating plan that will support your stomach, liver and colon for healthy weight loss. It will also help you to keep your blood sugar levels balanced. This part contains a healthy shopping list and meal plans. The final chapter in this part tells you about natural food supplements.

The appendices give you the summary of motivational statements, Glycemic Index, guidelines for eating out, a savvy substitution list, recipes, and helpful resources. You'll also find a glossary, endnotes, bibliography, and index.

How to Use This Book

Start by reading chapter 1 on why diets fail. Then stop and take the assessment for your stomach, colon and liver in chapter 2. The next nine chapters list common imbalances that cause weight gain. Start with the chapter that interests you. Each chapter lists symptoms for each imbalance. Recommended tips and supplements listed in the chapter will help you to regain balance. Don't feel that you have to do *everything* listed in every chapter. That may be too overwhelming. If you have several areas you want to work on, I would suggest only taking one or two supplements or suggestions from each chapter.

Then go on to Part Eight, which puts it all together with an eating plan that is generally acceptable for any type of imbalance with a few exceptions that I mention in the book.

Give it a Chance!

No matter what you have tried, I encourage you to follow the ideas outlined in this book. I believe there are no impossible cases and that everyone can lose weight naturally and safely. Remember, weight loss is primarily a health issue.

Never Mind!

My identical twin sister, Jackie, is a woman of faith and has been a great encouragement to me. When things go wrong, she says, "Never mind. Things can change." And they usually do!

So never mind how many chocolate eclairs you gobbled up at the office this morning. Never mind that you drool over rich pastries and tend to eat everything in sight when you feel depressed or stressed out. You can change! You can eat the right foods for your body, you can resist temptation, and you can lose weight and keep it off.

Excess body fat disappears when the body is working properly. Whether you want to lose ten, fifty, or one hundred pounds, you can safely achieve your goal by learning to eat the right kinds of foods for your body. I believe we can all win the "No-Belly" prize!

Everyone can win over weight! I can and will lose weight safely. Forget the past—it's a new day!

PART ONE

No More Fad Diets

My people are destroyed for lack of knowledge.
Hosea 4:6

Chapter One

Forget Dieting!

When I first began studying about whole foods and cooking in the mid-70s, breadmaking was my favorite class to teach. I had a wheat grinder to grind wheat berries. Every Tuesday my house was filled with the aroma of freshly baked whole-wheat bread. By the end of the evening, my tummy was filled with freshly baked whole-wheat bread!

My Weight Kept Finding Me!

Even though I was eating healthier foods, I was still overweight. I found myself trying various diets that came along. I might lose a few pounds here and there, but they never stayed off. The weight I lost kept finding me—that is, until I learned the principles shared in this book. After years of fad dieting, I have learned that the only things quick and instant are microwaves, credit cards, and coffee!

Why Are We Still Overweight?

In spite of all of our efforts to lose weight, the diet industry does a whopping thirty-billion-dollar business annually.

Why? Because ninety-five out of one hundred of those who lose weight by dieting, gain it right back! We don't need another diet—we need a healthy lifestyle and an understanding of how our bodies work.

Obesity Is Risky

Millions of Americans are currently overweight. If you are overweight your risk for cancer, heart disease, and diabetes increases dramatically. Even high cholesterol and high blood pressure are connected with obesity.

Dieting Makes Us Fat

We need to take charge of our own health, but fad diets don't work. If they did, you and I probably would have been slender and healthy after the first diet we tried. According to Bob Schwartz, in his book *Diets Still Don't Work,* there have been as many as 26,000 diets.[1] I've had many clients who remained fat because they started to fad diet! This is called "diet-induced" obesity or weight-gain because of dieting. In order to better understand the futility of fad diets, let's look at the reasons why they fail.

Mental Trap. *"Be ye transformed by the renewing of your mind"* (Rom. 12:2).

People think that overweight people must lack discipline. "Otherwise," they reason, "why else would they be overweight?" But this statement is not always true. In the past ten years I've worked with hundreds of clients struggling with weight problems. In that time, I've discovered that many people simply lack the knowledge as to how to eat healthy. In many instances their bodies are out of balance, which causes food cravings. Most overweight people eat the wrong foods in the wrong way and therefore are not cooperating with their fat-burning ability. As a result, they lack energy. I'm far more disciplined when I have energy—aren't you?

Everyone Has Discipline!

Once these people change their eating habits, the weight comes off. I encourage my clients to get off the dieting merry-go-round and to use the discipline and energy they do have, to eat in such a way as to nourish, and re-balance the body so it can burn fat properly. In other words, my plan "cooperates" with the way the body was originally designed.

Dieting starts a cycle that looks like this:

- setting an unrealistic goal
- planning a quick diet
- experiencing stress and frustration
- binging and then starting all over again

Like a merry-go-round, dieting causes your life to be centered around food. When I was in the diet trap, I was busy writing my list of "foods to eat" while other people were writing their lists of "things to do." Dieting, I learned, is a temporary answer with temporary results. Consequently, for short periods of time I was slim—over and over again!

Wrong Expectations

Another part of the mental trap is the unrealistic expectations put on women and that women put on themselves. What causes this unrealistic image? Why do women try an endless array of fad diets to get down to an often unrealistic weight, only to regain it again? Advertisements, movies, and TV show models whose lifestyles are about staying in shape. The average model is 5'9" and weighs 123 pounds. Yet eighty-five percent of American women are 5'4" and weigh 144 pounds. Only one in forty thousand women has a model's body. Rather than try to have a model's body, it's more realistic and natural to let your body find its own natural shape.

Men have often been taught to expect women to look like models, and can put unrealistic demands on girlfriends or spouses. Conversely, there are equal expectations for American men to bulk up, looking like Green Bay linebackers with massive biceps and trim waists.

Now I Feel Great!

Get healthy first and the weight loss will follow. Chris, one of my clients, recently said: "I first came to see Lorrie for weight loss. I felt so much better and had so much more energy after following her advice that I didn't worry so much about the weight loss. But I did lose weight too!"

Emotional Trap. *"And he shall give you another Comforter, that he may abide with you forever"* (John 14:16).

For many people with a "diet mentality" food is their comforter. Eating high-sugar, processed foods can soothe emotional pain. Since food was not meant to comfort us emotionally, people with this mindset can never get enough food.

Also, dieting usually means we eat foods we don't like, so we don't find dieting enjoyable. The diet trap causes us to label foods "good" and "bad" and attaches an emotion as we eat them. I've known some dieters to order ice cream by saying, "I'll have a bowl of guilt ripple!"

But I Want M&M's!

Simply labeling foods "good" and "bad" can cause cravings. The more we are told not to eat a certain food, the more we want it. Take M&M's for instance. They are high in fat and sugar and contain little nutrition. Ants ignore them on a picnic, attacking your chicken sandwich instead!

When we finally give in to the lure of M&M's, we don't eat one or two, but devour the whole bag—and not even taste them!

My Tummy Hurts!

There's a difference between knowing by experience that something isn't good for you (you had a stomachache after eating it), and having someone tell you that something is not good for you. I recently had a client say to me, "Lorrie, I feel so much better when I don't drink coffee." I had suggested some time ago that she eliminate coffee. When *she* took the initiative to change, and when *she* experienced better health, the results were effective and the change was permanent.

Most diets are based on the "do this, don't do that" principle. The Life Design plan is based on teaching you to make wise food choices, based on good health.

Ummm, Good!

Most Americans eat certain foods because they taste good, never mind that they may be toxic to your body. In this book, you'll gain a new perspective about foods, based not on taste but on results.

Health Is Our First Goal

Another part of emotional eating is this: you cannot separate your mind and body. Make health your first goal. When you eat better, you think and feel better. (However, I respect licensed counselors and never hesitate to refer a client to one if emotional counseling seems necessary.)

Social Trap. *"Prove all things; hold fast that which is good"*
(1 Thess. 5:21).

Dieting is not natural. The hardest part about dieting is not watching what you eat, but what others eat. If you have ever eaten carrot sticks while your friends ate lasagna, you know what I mean.

Food Is Everywhere

Once I went three months without eating sweets, except for one fateful night at a writer's club banquet. "One piece won't hurt," I rationalized, choosing the biggest piece of cheesecake. It was delightful. Just moments earlier, I had arrived at the banquet full of self-control. By the end of the evening, I was full of cheesecake! Whether it's a banquet or a party, celebrations are a part of life.

We'll always have opportunities to blow it. I had to train myself to learn how to eat so I didn't gain weight every time I ate out. Part of learning how to stay healthy is learning to make good food choices even while dining out.

Spiritual Trap. *"For we wrestle not against flesh and blood"* (Eph. 6:12).

Dieting ignores the underlying spiritual problem behind the wrong foods and wrong amounts, eaten at wrong times. You can starve your body through low-calorie dieting, but it won't do any permanent good. You will regain the weight until you deal with the deceptions, traps, and "triggers" that cause you to overeat. There must be a reason why I never chose to snack on an apple while watching the late news. Doritos always sounded better. If it were strictly a physical problem, like growing apples that tasted like Doritos, American ingenuity would have solved it by now.

It's All the Same Battle

The battle with temptation is the same whether it's a battle against alcohol, cigarettes, drugs, or food. We are coping with our problems through a substance.

I believe in prayer. I pray with my clients and my staff, and I pray for my clients daily. However, many people attempt to make changes mentally and spiritually without changing *physically*, too. It's hard, for example, to pray and fast when your body is fatigued or toxic. If you've ever felt dizzy, tired and weak while trying to fast, you know it's no fun.

Does it Really Matter?

Throughout the years, I've had many people ask, "Aren't we just supposed to pray and expect God to bless our food? Does it really matter *what* we eat?"

If all God wanted was for us to pray, then why even teach about nutrition? Why even have nutritionists or doctors for that matter? Why not just pray about everything? Would you ever put the wrong fuel in your gas tank and then just pray that your car would run properly? No, your car needs the right fuel, or it won't run. So does your body. We are responsible to care for our bodies, and that includes choosing and eating healthy foods.

Although this book will focus on the physical aspects of weight loss, I recommend getting spiritual counseling if you need it.

Physical Trap. *"Be ye not unwise . . ."* (Eph. 5:17).

This book is about the nutritional reasons for diet failures, so let's look at a few popular diets and see why they fail.

Low-Calorie Diets

For years, most people accepted the idea that low-calorie diets were the only way to lose weight. But for many of us on low-calorie diets, the only things we ever lost were hope and money! Unfortunately, low-calorie diets do not result in permanent weight loss. On the contrary, they set the stage for a continual pattern of gaining and losing weight. Yo-yo dieting has been linked to gallbladder problems, heart disease, and a slower rate of metabolism.

The Bottom Line

Everyone remembers when Oprah Winfrey lost sixty-seven pounds on a four-hundred-calories-a-day liquid diet. When she came off the diet and ate solid foods again, she immediately regained thirty pounds. Low-calorie dieting fails because it teaches your body to store fat.

When you stop eating, your body reacts as if you are starving, and it slows down your metabolism—your fat-burning ability. Pounds drop at first, but later your body slows down and fights your intention to keep dropping those pounds. When you start eating again, you gain weight because of your slower metabolism. So you always gain more on low-calorie diets.

Your body becomes much more efficient at storing fat (in case there is a famine!). So after you regain the weight, it takes longer to lose it the second time around. Actually, you gain faster and faster.

Achieving permanent weight loss means consuming less calories and fats than you normally do, while eating enough to still stay healthy. This means eating nutrient-dense foods, or foods that pack much more nutrition per calorie. Our body is sensitive to the nutrition in food, not the volume of food.

High-Protein Diets

Examples of high-protein diets are the Atkins, Protein Power and Stillwell. These diets emphasize a high-protein consumption (more than one hundred grams a day), usually of animal foods with low or no carbohydrates.

The main benefit of this diet is that it addresses the problem of sugar cravings. People lose sugar cravings because they don't stimulate the release of the "hunger" hormone, insulin. Their blood sugar level is stable because they eat few if any carbohydrates. However, many of my clients who strictly followed this diet and went off the diet, lost the symptomatic relief gained. Because our bodies need some carbohydrates to make the chemicals in the brain to reduce cravings, this diet can set up binges. I've had clients who even went from eating high-protein foods for weeks, to binging on cookies and ice cream!

Physical Imbalances

Here are some problems I've seen with clients who followed a high-protein diet, but failed to take into account possible deficiencies this diet may cause:

- The high-protein diet is high in Omega 6 (animal) fats. Since most of my clients are deficient in Omega 3 fats, this diet can aggravate an essential fat deficiency. (See chapter 14.)
- The high-protein diet increases the need for additional protease (a digestive enzyme) necessary for proper protein digestion. Many of my clients, already deficient in these enzymes, found they were even further deficient following this diet. (Enzymes are discussed in chapter 3.)
- I've observed that for some of my clients, the high-protein diet aggravates PMS/menopausal symptoms. (See chapter 11.)
- The high-protein diet further aggravates the vital need for proper vitamins and minerals, which many of my clients were deficient in. Additionally, plant foods high in phytochemicals so necessary for preventing cancer, are minimized in this diet. (See chapter 17.)
- Since many of my clients were not getting enough fiber, this diet, low in fiber, increases the risk of constipation, hemorrhoids and other colon problems. (See chapter 13.)
- Finally, many of my clients didn't know to eat high-quality proteins, and fats. Processed meats can contain nitrates and other cancer-causing chemicals. (See chapter 15.)

I've observed the faces of clients who have stayed on the high-protein diet for a time. Often they came in with pale skin and bags under their eyes. I've helped these clients detox their kidneys and liver and enjoy a more balanced approach to eating. They look and feel much better.

Additionally women with high levels of estrogen should never follow a high-animal protein diet—nor should people with kidney disease or osteoporosis.

High-Carbohydrate Diet

The high-carbohydrate diet emphasizes whole grains, beans and legumes, and is usually low in animal protein. Chinese and Indian people do well on this diet. However, for many others, and especially women over forty, a diet like this can be too high in starches, which can lead to food cravings and weight gain. (For a greater understanding of why this diet may have failed, see chapters 10 and 13.)

Carbohydrate, Fat or Protein-Restricted Diets

Balance is essential for a healthy body, and all elements are required. Eating the right kind of carbohydrates is important. Likewise, a small amount of the right type of fat can actually increase your fat-burning potential! And protein is required daily. So be cautious about any diet that eliminates any of these important elements.

Unhealthy Stimulants

Taking artificial stimulants can damage the heart, adrenals, central nervous system, and metabolism. Fenphen and Redux were proven to have serious side effects. The sad truth is that once the drugs are stopped, the weight-loss effects stop as well. No permanent lifestyle changes are made. Relying on drugs alone, without taking responsibility for making lifestyle changes is sure to fail. In addition, stimulants fail to get to the root of the health problems that cause obesity.

We've seen the disastrous results of taking these drugs. I've often wondered, did the people who used the products think to read the warnings on the package inserts that come with such drugs?

Even "natural" stimulants like caffeine, ma huang, and guarana can be damaging to the heart and adrenal glands when used over long periods of time. (More details on this subject in chapter 6.) And drinking too many "diet" teas that contain large amounts of senna can cause the body to lose important nutrients.

Surgeries

Another popular, quick weight-loss method is surgery. Whether it's wiring the jaw, stapling the stomach, liposuction, or tummy tucks, once the surgery is over, the person is often still the same. Unless lifestyle changes are made and unless changes are made to enhance the body's fat-burning ability, the weight problem will probably still be there. After spending all that money, this can be discouraging.

Conventional Diets

Conventional diet centers can help people with portion control, behavioral modification, and lifestyle changes, but most conventional diets fail to look at the nutritional issues. Diet plans won't help if the body is nutritionally out of balance. Any plan that doesn't help to eliminate cravings or hunger by working with the body's natural design, is doomed to fail. Most of these cravings fall away when the nutritional deficiencies are addressed.

A client whom we'll call Melanie, was part of a diet program where she purchased prepared foods. She was spending several hundred dollars a month on pre-packaged foods and never lost weight. Tests that I conducted in my office revealed she was extremely deficient in enzymes. She never would have lost weight on that program no matter how careful and diligent she was to follow the plan. On my plan, Melanie has already lost twenty-five pounds!

Most diet plans fail because they don't address the individual or cooperate with how the body is designed. Our bodies are all different. There's no such thing as a "one diet fits all."

Meal Replacements

You may be surprised to discover that many of the liquid or powder meal-replacement drinks and food bars are nutritionally lacking and loaded with harmful ingredients. They don't address the hidden causes of overweight, the individuality of each person, or why certain "fat-free" foods actually hinder weight loss.

Clinical Nutrition

Designed clinical nutrition means working with your body, to determine your nutritional deficiencies and imbalances. Nutrition-minded health professionals such as Certified Nutritionists (C.N.), Clinical Certified Nutritionists (C.C.N.), Certified Nutrition Specialist (C.N.S.), Registered Dieticians (R.D.) nutrition-minded doctors (M.D. or D.O.), Naturopathic Doctors (N.D.), and chiropractors (D.C.) can use nutrition to balance your body.

Throughout this book, we'll be looking at various nutritional imbalances. Please don't self-diagnose. If you suspect a serious problem, see your doctor.

Our Goal Is Health

You probably didn't need to read this chapter to know that fad diets don't work; perhaps now you better understand why. Armed with that knowledge, you're ready to get started.

Next we'll discuss the top three causes for being overweight. You may be surprised!

I don't need to diet any more. I can eat the right foods to make me healthy. I'm ready to get healthy and lose weight safely.

Chapter Two

Take This Simple Test

It's hard to hide certain things. Back when I had an unlisted dress size, I wouldn't have been caught dead in a pair of jeans! Sometimes it seems appropriate to conceal things. However, when it comes to weight loss, we need the truth. Why do people struggle with weight? Obviously, we need to "eat less and exercise more." But what about the people who do eat less and exercise more, yet never lose weight?

Fat Thighs Forever?

Many people come to my office feeling guilty about their weight problem. After they've tried everything, it's only normal to feel frustrated. When I was overweight, I remember looking at my fat thighs and feeling doomed to live with them forever. When I was a compulsive overeater, I couldn't even imagine myself thin, because I craved food so much! Since that time, I've learned a great deal about my body and the health issues. So take hope! There are answers.

Weight Problems Are Health Problems

There is a definite relationship between what we eat and how we feel. I've seen this cause-and-effect relationship in the area of weight loss, too.

Before I went into private practice, I taught weight-loss classes and counseled people for eight years, always stressing the importance of proper digestion. In the past two years, I have privately counseled hundreds of clients who now enjoy more energy and safe weight loss. When a client comes to my office for nutritional consultation, I *still* begin with their digestion. If food is not digested properly, the body cannot possibly process everything properly, sabotaging weight loss. Improper digestion can cause hunger and food cravings. So let's check your tummy out!

Check the Following:

Scan the following list and check (✔) the ones that apply to you. How many of these symptoms do you have?

- ☐ 1. Do you ever burp after meals?
- ☐ 2. Do you get stomachaches?
- ☐ 3. Do you overeat regularly?
- ☐ 4. Do you need to take an antacid after every meal?
- ☐ 5. Do you have indigestion regularly?
- ☐ 6. Do you often have heartburn or reflux?
- ☐ 7. Do you have gas or bloating after meals?
- ☐ 8. Do you have constipation or diarrhea?
- ☐ 9. Do you experience fatigue after eating?
- ☐ 10. Do you suffer from allergies?
- ☐ 11. Do you have dark circles under your eyes?
- ☐ 12. Do you have greasy or poorly-formed stools?

If you have even one of these symptoms, you may have tummy trouble! I've found that many health problems stem from poor digestion, especially obesity. Chapter 3 will get you on the road to better digestion and weight loss.

How About Your Colon?

The second area I address with clients is their colon. It's not what we eat, but what we absorb and assimilate that matters. Ideally, we should have regular bowel movements. If you are constipated, this may be contributing to your struggle with losing weight.

Check the Following:

Let's start with a colon check-up. Here are some common symptoms of colon problems. Check (✔) the ones that apply to you.

- ☐ 1. Do you suffer from chronic constipation?
- ☐ 2. Do you have a bloated, distended, tender or rigid abdomen?
- ☐ 3. Do you have regular gas and flatulence?
- ☐ 4. Do you suffer from colitis?
- ☐ 5. Do you have poor circulation?

❐   6. Are you overweight?

❐   7. Do you have chronic lower-back pain?

❐   8. Do you have bad breath?

❐   9. Do you have bad body odor (feet, hands, under arms)?

❐ 10. Do you have frequent headaches?

❐ 11. Do you have a poor appetite or abnormal cravings for food?

❐ 12. Do you have skin problems or acne?

If you checked even one or two of these symptoms, you may need to do a colon cleanse. Chapter 4 will tell you how and why.

How's Your Liver?

The third and most important area is the functioning of your liver, your key organ for fat metabolism. Proper liver function can help your body to increase its natural ability to burn fat.

Our bodies are continually cleansing and eliminating wastes through the liver, gallbladder, kidneys, gastrointestinal tract, and skin. Unfortunately, the type and amounts of foods we eat can be too much for our body to process. Especially in America where there's a restaurant or grocery store on every corner!

Overeating is so common. Our liver was designed to detoxify our body's waste. However, in recent years, the liver has been called on to do extra duty. It now has to filter out extra toxins from pollution, additives, preservatives, coffee, sodas, junk foods, and excesses. This puts stress on the liver, demanding it to do things it was never designed to do.

Think about the filter on your furnace or air conditioning unit. When it gets full, we take it out and clean it. Well, often we eat foods and drink beverages that overload the liver, hindering its efforts at metabolizing fats. When was the last time you cleansed your liver? Most people, especially those with weight problems, never do cleanse their liver, but they should. Think of it this way: the liver has a very long "to do" list, and fat burning is at the bottom!

Check the Following:

These symptoms may indicate a sluggish liver. Check (✔) the ones that apply to you.

☐   1. Do you have a hormonal imbalance (both men and women)?
☐   2. Do you suffer from moodiness, irritability, and confusion?
☐   3. Do you have PMS (irregular menstrual cycle, cramps, or breast tenderness)?
☐   4. Do you have bloating?
☐   5. Do you have high cholesterol?
☐   6. Do you have eye problems?
☐   7. Do you have a coated tongue?
☐   8. Do you have bad breath?
☐   9. Do you have problems with low-blood sugar?
☐ 10. Do you get chilled after a meal?
☐ 11. Do you have headaches frequently?
☐ 12. Do you have an eating disorder?
☐ 13. Do you have skin diseases and problems (including pigment on the back of hands)?
☐ 14. Do you have nausea frequently?
☐ 15. Do you have frequent allergies?
☐ 16. Do you have constipation and/or diarrhea?

Well, how did you do? If you checked one or two of the preceding questions, your liver needs nutritional support. Chapter 5 will help you.

How Did We Get This Way?

Nutritionist, Dr. Lindsey Duncan, says, "Under ideal circumstances, the body is well equipped to neutralize and dispose of toxins through the liver, spleen and eliminative channels (bowel, kidneys, lungs, skin and lymphatic system). But in modern day society there are no ideal circumstances." Duncan further states,

> Our digestive system is the most abused. We've been raised on a diet of bread, dairy, cheese, meat, fast foods, fried foods, fatty foods, sweets, candy, ice cream, etc. Over time these foods break down the digestive and eliminative system, causing fatigue, gas, bloating, poor

elimination, poor digestion, poor skin, brain fog, low-blood sugar, etc. ...the end result of foods that aren't broken down properly and waste by-products that aren't eliminated properly. We must not let trapped toxins and wastes pollute our bloodstream and the rest of our organs! Digestive inefficiency can continue even after dietary improvements if you don't help rejuvenate your intestinal system through internal cleansing.[1]

What Can You Expect?

Processed foods mentioned above actually break down the digestive system. Part Two will help you support your digestive system. Here's what you can expect from improving your digestion:

- Safe weight loss
- Better digestion
- Improved elimination
- More energy
- Less cravings
- Fewer or no headaches
- No more depression

I no longer need to stay the way I am. Things seen are about to change!

What Are the Top Three Causes of Weight Gain?

Bring to light the hidden things...
1 Corinthians 4:5

Chapter Three

How's Your Tummy?

We often feel we can eat anything we like because fat doesn't instantly show up on our legs and arms, and our tummies don't extend immediately. Give it time. Because we eventually do reap what we sow!

We *Can* Eat Anything

The issue is not what we are eating, but what happens to the food after it's eaten. The foods we eat today create the blood and/or nourishment we use tomorrow, which results in the condition of our health—whether good or bad.

Americans pop digestive aids like candy and spend millions of dollars a year on laxatives and antacids; yet they continue to suffer from poor digestion and elimination. If these products really "fixed" the problem, why do we still need them? What's the real problem?

In his book, *The Mysterious Cause of Illness,* Dr. Jonn Matsen explains that our stomachs "harden" in response to eating and drinking certain substances.[1] We then think we can eat anything, because we seem to get away with it for a time. Sooner or later, however, digestive problems surface. Here's what happens. When we first drink something unnatural, such as coffee, our alarm sounds loud and clear—perhaps we'll have a stomachache. But if we repeatedly override that natural alarm, after a while the body gives up its warning signals and adapts to the stress. Your amazing stomach quits complaining and says, "Okay, have it your way then!" You think you feel better after a cup of coffee because of the stimulation.

Your body won't talk to you again until the symptoms are much more serious—an ulcer for example. Uh-oh! Too late!

WHAT HURTS YOUR TUMMY?

If you were raised in the States, you were probably raised on the typical American diet. Here's a list of several factors that can cause poor stomach functioning:

- Eating too many fatty foods
- Eating white sugar and artificial sugar substitutes
- Eating refined, processed, cooked foods and refined carbohydrates (candy, cookies, cake, etc.)
- Eating fried foods
- Drinking too much caffeine
- Not getting enough fiber
- Overuse of antacids
- Excess red meat consumption
- Drinking alcohol or smoking
- Eating too fast
- Poor chewing
- Overeating
- Stress

A major goal of this book is to help you strengthen your ability to digest food and lose weight. The stronger your digestive system, the better your health. The better your health, the easier your weight loss!

How Digestion Works

The stomach is the first stage of digestion. As your stomach mixes food, it releases acidic digestive juices, which help break down foods. I have found that as people improve their digestion, they find weight loss easy and natural. Food cravings and hunger are closely linked to digestive problems.

What's a Digestive Enzyme?

Enzymes are a type of protein that help to digest, absorb, transport, metabolize, and eliminate waste.

One of the most important jobs of enzymes is to digest our food, making it so small that it can pass through the minute openings of the intestines into the bloodstream.

When Esther first came to my office, she complained of stomach problems. When I asked her if she'd ever taken enzymes, she gave me a blank look and replied, "What are enzymes?" and "What can they do for me?"

Her response is not uncommon. I've met few clients who understand what enzymes are or how they help digestion. Esther's stomach problems are almost gone since she began taking digestive enzymes. Let's see why.

If you are eating a balanced diet, getting enough exercise and sleep, taking vitamins, and you still don't feel energetic, you may lack digestive enzymes.

How Do Enzymes Help?

Good enzyme supplements are wonderful for improving digestion, but they also contribute to other health benefits:

BENEFITS OF ENZYMES

- Aid digestion
- Boost your energy
- Boost metabolism
- Detoxify
- Slow aging
- Aid in weight loss
- Aid in a faster response from injury and inflammation

Types of Enzymes

Our bodies contain literally thousands of enzymes. The most common of these are:

Protease

Protease digests protein. After taking them, most people notice a decrease in symptoms of gas, constipation, or indigestion. Protease can also digest certain bacteria and viruses. And proteolytic enzymes are also used for inflammation associated with arthritis and sports injuries. Generally, signs of inflammation and pain are reduced with these enzymes.

Amylase

Amylase digests carbohydrates, and is quite helpful for people who have trouble digesting complex carbohydrates. Amylase is an enzyme that can help diabetics to handle sugars and starches. It also helps with skin problems like psoriasis and eczema.

Lipase

Lipase digests fats and fat-soluble vitamins. Many overweight people are deficient in this enzyme. Lipase can help prevent high cholesterol and triglycerides, weight gain, and heart disease, and is a supportive enzyme for the liver and gallbladder.

Lactase

Lactase is an enzyme that breaks down milk sugar. If you've "got milk" but also "got" bloating, gas, or diarrhea, you probably have lactose intolerance. Avoid dairy products, or take a lactase enzyme.

How Are Enzymes Destroyed?

All cooked foods totally lack enzymes! Enzymes are heat sensitive, so cooking foods over 118°F. destroys these vital enzymes. This includes cooking, baking, frying, and microwaving. Cooking doesn't improve the nutritional value of food. It destroys or makes unavailable 85 percent of the original nutrients.

Less Enzymes Means More Fat!

Most Americans live on a diet that is 99 percent cooked foods completely free from enzymes. The average family spends as little as $1 or $2 a week on fresh produce. Eating plenty of raw foods takes the stress off the endocrine system. A diet of cooked foods causes glands to become over-stimulated. This causes oversecretion of hormones, overeating, and obesity.

Your Enzyme Bank Account

We are born with a certain number of enzymes or an enzyme bank. Using up our digestive enzymes hinders our ability to make metabolic enzymes. That means we are pulling on our "reserves," and once these are gone—well, let's put it this way—we're gone! The body calls on enzymes from other parts of the body to finish the job. This can weaken your body and make it vulnerable to disease.

Replenish Your Account

Does this mean we have to throw away our pots and pans and live entirely on raw fruits and vegetables? No. Like my friend Catherine says,

"Your family may not be ready for raw asparagus soup!" If you can't eat plenty of raw foods, you need to replenish your enzymes, or add enzyme deposits to your account. I'll tell you how later in this chapter.

Enzyme Deficiencies Are Everywhere!

In his book, *Self-Test Nutrition Guide,* Dr. Cass Ingram reports that:

> ...enzyme deficiency is extremely common in the United States as well as in other Western countries. . . . the pancreas fails to produce the appropriate amount of enzymes for foods to be digested optimally . . . largely a result of enzyme burnout from the prolonged consumption of processed and chemically contaminated foods.[2]

Dr. Ingram goes on to state that nearly 80 percent of the calories consumed by Americans today come from processed foods. There are well over 6,000 synthetic chemicals, which are "legally" added to food. It's no wonder that pancreatic disease is common in America today.[3]

Ingram lists substances that hurt the pancreas such as: coffee, alcohol, tobacco, smoke, artificial sweeteners, food preservatives, food dyes, drugs, sulfites, MSG, pesticides, herbicides, and refined sugar. He adds that a high-sugar diet will cause a significant reduction in pancreatic enzyme output.[4]

In addition to refined white sugar, Ingram warns about the use of artificial sweeteners, which may cause toxicity to the pancreas. He writes, "Studies document that NutraSweet essentially stops the pancreas from producing enzymes."[5] That's a pretty sober warning!

Do You Need Enzymes?

On the next page is a list of criteria you might want to consider to determine if you need enzyme supplements:

YOU NEED ENZYMES IF YOU ...

- are not eating plenty of raw fruits and vegetables
- are overweight
- are diabetic
- overeat regularly
- are under stress
- have bowel or digestive problems
- drink coffee or sodas
- eat white sugar, candy, cakes, and cookies often
- eat only cooked and processed foods

How Can I Get Enzymes?

There are only three ways to restore your vital enzyme bank:

1. Eat more raw fruits and vegetables.
2. Buy a juicer and juice fresh fruits and vegetables. Have at least one glass every day.
3. Take a supplemental enzyme formula.

A well-balanced supplement will contain protease, amylase, lipase, pancreatin, and/or betaine hydrochloric acid (see next section). Enzyme supplements are safe, and they can even help reduce your need for certain vitamin and mineral supplementation.

Your health food store carries several enzyme formulas. Here are a few: Super Digestaway by Solary, Megazyme by Enzymatic Therapy (has HCl), Nature's Secret Multiple Enzymes, Multizyme by Nature's Life, Super Enzyme Caps by Twin Lab, Ultrazyme by Nature's Plus, Enzymes by Michael's, or Daily Enzyme Formula by Prevail. For digesting beans, try Beano or Say Yes to Beans by Nature's Plus. Try Say Yes to Dairy for digesting dairy products. In my office I use a professional type of enzymes called Zypan (with HCl) or Multizyme (without HCl) by Standard Process. See Appendix J for a number to call to find a health professional near you who carries Standard Process supplements.

Hydrochloric Acid

In addition to enzymes, your stomach also makes hydrochloric acid, or HCl, for breaking down protein. Americans start to have deficiencies of HCl at an average age of thirty-five to forty-five. This condition is known as hypochlorhydria, and it affects half of the people over age fifty. Lack of HCl leads to many problems such as: constipation, flatulence, and cramps. Today, even teenagers are showing a deficiency of this important nutrient. Why? Again, blame it on processed foods.

HCl is important because it's vital for the digestion of proteins. Also, HCl stimulates the gallbladder to secrete bile needed for fat metabolism. When bile secretion is insufficient due to lack of HCl, proper fat metabolism is impaired. The bottom line—no weight loss!

SYMPTOMS OF HCl DEFICIENCY
• Bad breath
• Bloating and gas
• Cramping
• Constipation
• Passage of undigested food
• Belching
• Coated tongue

Antacid Addiction

Americans spend two billion dollars a year on antacids! Full-page advertisements for people with heartburn report that "Some two hundred and thirty-seven million prescriptions have been written for Tagamet."[6]

Antacids are called the "most prescribed medication of its kind" boasting of 550 million consumers. That adds up to an incredible number of people with sour stomachs!

But Tagamet, or any antacid, is not the answer to the problem because it never gets to the root cause. Unfortunately, commercial antacids in wafers, powders, or bicarbonate of soda actually decrease the supply of HCl and add to digestive trouble!

Long-term overuse of antacids is one of the reasons why many people suffer from ulcers. As Dr. Lindsey Duncan once said, "Poor digestion is not a Rolaids deficiency!"

Too Much or Too Little?

Without enough HCl, a protein meal not well-digested stays in the stomach. Chemical reactions produce an acid that causes heartburn and bloating. So you take Tums or some other antacid. However, this "acid indigestion" may be caused by *not enough* HCl! Both insufficient *and* excess HCl produce the same symptoms. How can you tell the difference? Buy a good enzyme product with "betaine hydrochloride, pancreatin, and pepsin." (The one I carry is called Zypan. Your health food store will carry several brands.) If your symptoms improve, you have *low* HCl, and Zypan would help you. If they worsen, you need a good enzyme *without* HCl to rebalance your stomach acid. (I have used Gastrex or Gastrozyme very successfully with clients in my office. If you can't find a good enzyme that works, see a health professional who has experience with enzymes.)

Natural Health Drinks Restore HCl

There are two simple, inexpensive ways in which HCl can be added to your digestive system. Putting the juice of one half of a lemon in your water is one way. The second is drinking apple cider vinegar.

A common folk remedy for getting hydrochloric acid is to mix 1 teaspoon of apple cider vinegar and 1 teaspoon honey in an eight-ounce glass of water and drink upon arising.

Apple cider vinegar is an excellent source of HCl which will in turn assist with weight loss. Apple cider vinegar is a therapeutic vinegar for cleansing and alkalizing the system and is great for daily used in salads. (As an added bonus, apple cider vinegar has many other health benefits. See Appendix B for a listing of these benefits.)

Not all vinegar is the same. Purchase natural, *raw*, undistilled apple cider vinegar from a health food store. It's naturally fermented and fully aged in wooden barrels. Look for fully-ripened vinegars that have sediment floating in the bottom. Our grandmothers called this the "mother." It's the sign that it is truly fermented. Locate a natural source; otherwise, you're wasting your good money.

What Else Can I Do?

Early in my practice, I had several clients who faithfully took good digestive enzymes, but still had digestive problems. One client, Darlene, reported that only after she went to a chiropractor and had a certain adjustment, did she finally see an improvement with her digestion. Since then I've learned how vital proper chiropractic care is, and recommend that my clients consider chiropractic adjustments along with good nutrition.

How Do You Feel?

Are you full of energy or generally fatigued? One reason why you may feel fatigued is that your body is working overtime trying to digest too much food. When foods are eaten properly, it takes half the time and energy to digest, leaving you with much more energy (and time)!

Hundreds of years ago, people ate more simply. Our bodies weren't designed to adapt to modern meals and modern processing methods. Eating many different types of foods at one meal weakens the digestive tract, which can cause all kinds of tummy trouble. Poor digestion and poor assimilation cause proteins to putrefy, fats to become rancid, and carbohydrates to ferment—right in your body!

BENEFITS OF FOOD COMBINING

1. Aids digestion, which increases available energy and enhances overall health

2. Reduces stress on the entire digestive system

3. Reduces gas and bloating

4. Makes weight loss more efficient

5. Makes meal planning easier

A Missing Piece

Food combining is the process of eating specific foods that digest well together. I have been familiar with the idea of food combining for more than twenty years. Dozens of my clients have experienced marked improvement in their digestive function and their weight loss by following these principles. If you have great health and great metabolism, fine! Skip this section. But if weight loss is slow for you, read on. Stoke those digestive fires!

Here's a short list of starches and proteins so you will understand what we mean when we get to the food combining principles:

Complex Carbohydrates
Potatoes
Brown rice

Proteins
Eggs
Red meat

Complex Carbohydrates	**Proteins**
Whole grain breads	Cheese
Starchy vegetables	Fish
Whole-grain pastas	Turkey
Beans	Chicken
Oatmeal	Milk/dairy

Food Combining Principles

There are many books written about food combining, a subject which Harvey and Marilyn Diamond made popular in their book, *Fit for Life*. I've simplified these principles.

1.   Probably one of the most important guidelines is to eat fruits (raw and cooked) and other highly sweetened foods alone, preferably in the morning before other meals. Fruits are easily digested and become part of your bloodstream within an hour. However, by adding other concentrated foods like those listed in the complex carbohydrate and protein columns, the fruit ferments often causing gas. Improper food combining can cause a headache among other things. So eat your watermelon *first*, not after your chicken, potatoes and coleslaw.

By the way, the combination of starch, fruit, protein and sugar is hard to digest (such as candy, cakes and cookies) and especially bad is the combination of eggs, milk, and sugar (recognize ice cream?).

2.   Generally, proteins and carbohydrates are eaten separately, but I've found that eating lighter proteins like fish or chicken combine fairly well with a starch, like brown rice or a potato. Have one serving of each, not two servings of each! In other words, have some rice and a chicken Caesar salad. Period. And take your enzymes.

3.   You may want to eat your lobster and steak, or chicken and cheese entree together, but don't. According to experts, each of these proteins takes different enzymes, so you're better off just eating one protein at a time. It's worse when animal proteins are fried with cooking oils.

The goal is to strengthen your stomach, not weaken it. Concentrated proteins like meat and chicken also digest better in small amounts. Proteins combine best with vegetables, so a piece of chicken, fresh salad, and steamed vegetables would make a nice meal.

You don't need milk and protein at a meal, either. This means that a Big Mac and shake are really out! The best way to handle this kind of combination is if the milk is curdled, as with yogurt. (A Big Mac and vanilla yogurt? I doubt if that catches on!)

4.   You can combine different starches together since they require the same enzyme for digestion. This means you could eat brown rice and potatoes and starchy vegetables all at the same meal. But for most people, that can add up to too many starches.

What If You Eat Out Often?

What if you don't combine foods well or you eat out often? Take digestive enzymes! Complex carbohydrates combine well with vegetables. A nice meal would be whole-grain brown rice, chicken, and a salad or vegetables. Vegetables can be paired with either proteins or starches. One way to get these foods together in one meal is crockpot cooking. Slowly combining different foods like grains, vegetables, and animal meat in lots of water over a long time makes all of the foods in the crockpot easier to digest.

So trust me, your wonderful tummy is a key to your weight loss victory. This book will give you a way of eating to get that digestive spark going that causes an increase in metabolism, and that's your ticket to weight loss. Dr. Anthony Cichoke's book, *The Complete Book of Enzyme Therapy*, is one of the most comprehensive books on enzymes. Other good titles are listed in the Bibliography.

Nutritional Summary

- Take digestive enzymes
- Follow food-combining principles
- Take a Betaine Hydrochloride (or HCl) supplement
- Take a daily apple cider vinegar drink

Now I know how to eat to keep my tummy well. I love the foods that are good for me. Indigestion, heartburn, and sluggish metabolism are now a thing of the past.

Chapter Four

Me, Constipated?

Foreign invaders (toxic by-products) in the digestive track can wreak havoc on our weight-loss efforts. Amy was a health fitness trainer at the health club where my office was located. Tired, frustrated, and constipated, she came to me with questions about colon cleansing. She was in good shape, but she was constipated. And she couldn't get rid of her pouch no matter how many crunches she did. Bad breath was also a source of embarrassment to her. After cleansing her colon, her constipation, bad breath, and pouch were gone!

Toxic waste in a body with steel abs and toned thighs? All too possible. As a nutritionist and personal trainer, I've met dozens of clients with great bodies and toxic colons!

Your Digestive Hoover Vacuum Cleaner

The colon, or large intestine, is the end portion of the human digestive tract where waste is eliminated. The vacuum cleaner you use in your home draws in all the dust and dirt around the house. When the bag gets full you change it, right? Now think about your colon.

For years you have eaten food and assumed that, as though by magic, your body processed all good food, neutralized all the toxins, and just eliminated them. In a perfect world that might be true. Unfortunately, most of us don't have "Hoover colons!" In fact, if you have any kind of colon problem, like colitis, diverticulitis, or irritable bowel syndrome (IBS), it shows your colon has not been working properly.

One of my clients who had colon problems experienced relief from constipation simply by taking digestive enzymes. The first cause of any colon problem is lack of digestive enzymes, but there's more to it.

Prevention Is Better

Most Americans consume about seven to ten grams of fiber daily; a healthy number is twenty-five to thirty-five grams. In 1950, one in five Americans died of cancer of the colon, prostate or breast. In 1990, one in three people died. By the year 2000 it is predicted that one in two people will die of breast, prostate, or colon cancer. The sad fact is that many of these cancers can be prevented with healthy digestion and elimination.

Toxicity from the colon is not limited to the colon, because waste seeps into the bloodstream and to the rest of the body. I have long believed that the secret to long life, good looks, weight loss, and disease-free living is cleansing the colon.

Do You Need a Colon Sweep?

Colon problems are so rampant that in recent years Grandma's words, "Eat your roughage," have been making a comeback. Today we call it fiber. Did you know most of the food we eat lacks fiber? (Processed foods are again the culprit!) If we had been reared on a diet of fresh, whole foods, we would have had the fiber needed to clean toxic wastes out of our system. But since we didn't, we can help our body to sweep out those toxins by supplementing our diet with some kind of safe fiber. (I'll discuss how to get fiber later in this chapter.)

What Does My Colon Have to Do With Weight Loss?

You may still be wondering, why is a clean colon so important? Lack of fiber in the colon means that waste is not being eliminated properly. The walls of the colon can accumulate toxins. In fact many people have as much as ten pounds of old waste in their bowels. This is according to Dr. Bernard Jensen in his book, *Tissue Cleansing Through Bowel Management.* He further states, "In the 50 years I've spent helping people to overcome illness, disability, and disease, it has become crystal clear that poor bowel management lies at the root of most people's health problems."[1] Now that's something to think about!

Where Is the Build-Up?

Waste that cannot be eliminated has to go somewhere, right? But where? Some of it builds up on the colon walls (impacted feces, dead tissue, mucus, and even parasites) and the rest may block the digestive tract, which can cause constipation, weight gain, fatigue, and skin problems. An added bonus—many of my clients' chronic migraine headaches left following a good colon cleanse. Personally, I've noticed that when I keep my colon clean through eating well and a colon cleanse, I find I rarely need a deodorant. It's worth doing a spring cleaning in the colon, that's for sure!

Not in My Body!

Most people have no idea the kind of toxic waste that may accumulate in their colons. In fact, some health researchers believe that it could take up to a year to really clean the average colon. I've read that even if we are having three bowel movements a day, our colon still could be clogged.

I like how Dr. Lindsey Duncan puts it: "If you are eating three meals a day, and eliminating once, where are the other two meals?"[2]

The answer is, they are "hanging out" in your colon, waiting for some enzymes, fiber and water to push them along! Most people mistakenly think that one bowel movement per day is sufficient. The truth is less than two to three bowel movements a day is a sure sign of constipation.

Is Constipation Harmless?

People think of constipation as harmless. It is not. Constipation may be a warning sign of other more serious problems in the stomach, liver, or thyroid. Chronic constipation is serious and is linked to hemorrhoids, varicose veins, appendicitis, problems with the intestinal tract, and even cancer. Amy Steeves, a Certified Colon Hygienist from Houston who has done thousands of colonics stated in a recent interview:

> We have had clients who suffered from chronic constipation for 20 years who ended up with ovarian cancer. I'm not saying the constipation caused the cancer, but the buildup of accumulated toxins can cause them to seep through the colon wall. There is definitely a relationship.[3]

Our Body Parts Are Related

Robert Gray, author of *The Colon Health Handbook,* suggests that every point in the intestines is "reflexly" related to a specific body part. A toxic condition at one point of the intestinal tract can produce ill health in its reflexly-related body part.[4] For example, female problems in a woman may be related to some point in the colon that reflexes to her female organs. So, cleansing the colon may relieve these symptoms. In any case, there's no doubt that most everyone, especially those who grew up eating processed foods and unbalanced diets, can benefit from cleansing the colon. Earlier we said that lack of fiber causes some problems in the colon. What else causes colon problems? (See any processed foods in this list?)

WHAT HURTS THE COLON?

- A diet of white bread and refined foods
- Dairy products (milk and milk products)
- Over-cooked food
- Low-fiber foods
- Stress
- Regular use of antibiotics
- Prescription drugs
- B complex deficiency
- Consistent overeating
- Lack of exercise
- Lack of sufficient water
- Lack of essential fatty acids (good fats)
- Lack of "friendly" intestinal bacteria
- Lack of soluble and insoluble fiber

All of these hinder the colon from eliminating waste properly. Processed foods are like paste on your intestinal wall. Without fiber, this "paste" has nothing to move it out.

Try This!

Stir up a small mixture of flour and water in a paper cup and let it sit overnight. This will demonstrate the type of "paste" that clings to the walls of the intestines. Fiber is necessary to keep it moving.

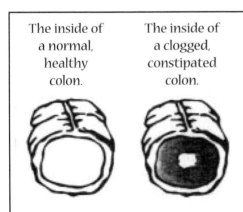

The inside of a normal, healthy colon.

The inside of a clogged, constipated colon.

The environment of the warm, dark, moisture-laden intestines is perfect for bacteria to grow and ferment. The by-product is acid that eats away at the intestinal lining, creating holes and sores. This is called Crohn's disease or colitis.

What Can I Do?

Colon elimination can be improved by eating a healthy diet, supplemented with good fiber and eliminative herbs, which we will look at shortly. However, if you want to do a serious colon cleanse, consider an enema or a colonic (similar to an enema but done privately with a Certified Colon Hygienist). You might be interested in knowing that in the early 1900s colonic machines were found in many doctors' offices, and even in hospitals. Unfortunately, drugs and surgery replaced some of these more natural approaches for healing.

Get Professional Help

Colonics (colon irrigation) and enemas both use purified water to flush out toxins from the bowel. Colonics, properly administered, are more thorough than enemas, but both help release colon waste. Steeves says: "The 'gravity flow' method of colon irrigation is the most natural. Prepackaged disposable nozzles and body drapes are used along with our state-of-the-art equipment. This method cleanses the colon by stimulating the natural action of the bowel. Using this type of colon irrigation is safe, gentle, and very effective. Warm, filtered water gently bathes the colon wall and can actually stimulate natural contractions of the bowel. Think of the gravity flow method as an exercise session for your colon."[5]

BENEFITS OF COLONICS:

- Colonics help to reshape the colon. Perhaps you have seen pictures of colons that have taken unusual shapes due to poor diet and lack of fiber. A properly administered colonic can help to reshape the colon and improve its function.
- Colonics help to remove impacted material on the colon wall.
- Colonics help to exercise the colon muscles. Peristaltic movement is the muscular contraction that moves material in the colon. Once the colon muscles are toned, this helps speed up the movement of material in the colon.
- Colonics help hydrate the body. Your body can absorb pure water to hydrate the cells of the body, which improves their function.

Herbal Support

Herbs have their place in colon cleansing, but they are not a substitute for colonics. Herbal laxatives undo the effects of temporary constipation, increase peristaltic contractions, and tone the colon. They are far safer than prescription and over-the-counter laxatives, which can be toxic. One client who came to me for help had used over-the-counter laxatives for more than ten years. This resulted in more serious health problems with her heart and she is still recovering.

Hang in There

Just one comment on this or any colon cleanse—drink lots of water and start slowly. You may experience diarrhea for a day or so, or even a mild headache while you detox. Stay with it. You'll be glad you did when you feel so much better. Today there are many natural products available to cleanse the colon. I recommend a colon cleanse at least twice a year.

Essiac—The Natural Wonder

Another great bloodstream cleanser is Essiac Tea, a cleansing tea that contains herbs that purify toxins in the bloodstream, lymph, colon and digestive tract. Not only will it help your colon, it is also very effective in eliminating cellulite!

Essiac is an effective, yet gentle detoxifier that cleanses body systems and organs. It was originally designed for cancer over sixty years ago and is well known as a cancer preventive. Even yeast sensitive people can use this formula.

A natural diuretic, it boosts the immune system, helps with constipation, purifies the blood and lymph, aids digestion and soothes the entire intestinal tract. For athletes, increases in endurance and strength are reported with decreased recuperation time. It's also an excellent skin moisturizer. Here is a short list of conditions which are helped: arthritis, asthma, allergies, cancer, Chronic Fatigue Syndrome, diabetes, irregularity, Parkinson's disease, swollen ankles, thyroid disorders, ulcers, urinary disorders varicose veins and warts.

Here are some common herbs that are contained in Essiac Tea.

Burdock Root is best know for its beneficial effect to the skin.
Sheep Sorrel is known for healing a wide variety of skin disorders.

It's been shown to strengthen the immune system and is rich in chlorophyll.

Turkish Rhubarb Root has been used in China more than 2,000 years. It has impressive detoxifying properties and is excellent liver cleanser with antibiotic and anti-microbial properties.

Cat's Claw has a great ability to cleanse the entire intestinal tract, boost immunity and decrease the pain and inflammation of arthritis.

Slippery Elm Root has been reported to reduce pain from ulcers because the mucilage coats any area it passes through. Also an antibiotic and anti-microbial, it helps remove toxins from the body.

I carry an excellent Essiac Tea and other colon cleansers. Your health food store carries other fiber cleansers and supplements.

Getting Fiber

By following the dietary suggestions in this book, you will be engaging in a "mild" colon cleanse just by eating higher-fiber foods. Good foods to help the colon include lentils, lightly steamed broccoli and cabbage, whole-grain brown rice, ginger, garlic and horseradish. (No, not all at once!) Sufficient fiber is vital to good health! The best source of fiber is the indigestible portion of foods, like the bran of grains and the pulp of fruits. It's good to get a variety of fibers and foods because they each contain different nutrients that aid other parts of the body. (See chapter 13 for easy ways to get more fiber.)

The best way to take a fiber supplement is to gradually begin with taking one teaspoon of oat bran, flaxseed, or psyllium seeds, (a type of natural fiber found in products such as Psyllium Wholehusks or powder or Nature's Plus Fiberitic Drink) and slowly increase the amount. After mixing the fiber in water, drink it quickly or it will become too thick to drink! Sometimes people become somewhat constipated when they first take a fiber supplement. This may be from a blocked or restricted area in the colon. This is why irrigating the colon is important to clear these blocked areas so the fiber can work better.

I recommend taking a fiber supplement that also contains some herbs for elimination and cleansing. The safest herbs are cascara sagrada and aloe vera. You can safely take three or four capsules at night—more if you don't have an elimination within a day. These herbs will help your bowels to move on their own.

Drink Plenty of Water

Be sure to drink eight to ten 8-ounce glasses of water to keep the plumbing operating! As you take the fiber and aloe vera supplements, decrease the amount of cascara until you have two to three daily regular bowel movements on your own. Other laxative-producing foods are prunes and prune juices. However, even if you use natural herbs like cascara, it is still necessary to eat a high-fiber diet, drink plenty of liquids, and exercise regularly.

More Good Guys

Another important food for colon health are the "friendly" bacteria. There are two types of bacteria living in your colon: friendly and unfriendly. Friendly bacteria on the colon wall help to break up food so the small villi that line the intestines can absorb food. The friendly bacteria are most commonly found in foods like yogurt, sourdough bread, sauerkraut, as well as miso and tempeh, which are soy-based cultured foods.

These friendly bacteria act as a natural antibiotic! People who have taken many antibiotics often lose this balance of friendly bacteria because the antibiotics kill both the bad and the good friendly bacteria. So in that case, it needs to be replaced by taking an acidophilus supplement of some kind. I've recommended these supplements to teenagers with skin problems, children with ear infections, and women with yeast infections. All were helped.

Americans are not accustomed to eating "cultured" foods, unless they like buttermilk (like my mother does) or natural yogurt. Not surprisingly, people in the countries where cultured foods are consumed have a lower incidence of colon cancers.

About Yogurt

Yogurt is a wonderful health food, but be sure to read labels and find one that says "contains live cultures." Most of the yogurt sold in grocery stores is loaded with sugar, additives and preservatives with hardly any real cultures.

The best solution is to take a supplement, often called probiotics or acidophilus. Nutrition NOW's PB8 or Prevail's Inner Ecology Powder can be found in a health food store. In my office, I use Lact-Enz or Lactic Acid Yeast by Standard Process and the Microbacs by Physician's

Choice. If you don't know a health professional, you can buy acidophilus supplements in health food stores, usually found in the refrigerator section.

An excellent book, *Cleansing Made Simple,* by Cheryl Townsley is a wonderful resource to learn more about cleansing.

Nutritional Summary

- Drink eight to ten 8-ounce glasses of water a day
- Get regular exercise
- Eat a healthy diet
- Take a fiber supplement
- Eat cultured foods or take an acidophilus supplement
- Do a colon cleanse at least twice a year
- Consider taking colonics

I love how good I feel when my bloodstream and colon are cleansed, and I eat healthy foods. It's worth the time it takes to cleanse my body!

Chapter Five

How's Your Liver?

Wouldn't it be great if we had a fat-burning gauge attached to our bodies like the thermostat in our homes? Then we could just turn it up whenever we wanted to burn more fat. Every American would buy one! We would crank it up after those gourmet meals that ended with chocolate mousse or lemon cheesecake, and turn it back when we regained consciousness! Welcome back to reality and to America—land of the professional gyms, spas, and weight-loss centers!

While you may not have such a gauge, you actually have more help than you may realize. For example, you already know that regular exercise increases the fat-burning ability. But did you know your liver holds a key to permanent weight loss?

Your Key to Weight Loss

I have learned a great deal from a Naturopathic Doctor in Seattle, Dr. Jonn Matsen, who regards *the liver as a vital organ for health and weight loss*. In his remarkable book, *The Mysterious Cause of Disease,* Matsen writes,

> ...since the liver is the main regulator of the blood, it is the true key to proper metabolic rate. A sluggish thyroid is often secondary to a long-term sluggish liver. Improving your digestion means improving the liver, which in turn improves the thyroid function.[1]

I have followed Dr. Matsen's suggestions for more than eight years and have found his advice to be true. When I help my clients improve their digestion and cleanse their liver and colon, weight loss is easier and usually permanent.

When Karen came to see me, she had unknowingly overburdened her liver. Her complaints were acne, constipation, fatigue and weight gain. Poor liver function was her primary cause of her problems. Following my six-week eating plan, Karen has lost twenty-five pounds. More importantly, her skin is clear and she is no longer fatigued. Your good health depends on the health of your liver.

Your Amazing Fat-Burning Organ

The more I study the liver, the more I am amazed at what it does! Research shows that the liver performs more than five hundred functions including: metabolize fats, proteins and carbohydrates, detoxify waste, filter the blood, store nutrients, manufacture bile, and regulate hormones and blood sugar.

Nearly everything the liver does is vital for proper weight management. Obviously, handling sugars and fats properly helps with fat loss and cravings. I've had client's who did everything right to lose weight, yet they never succeeded. I've found that if the liver is sluggish, no matter how much they work out, they can't lose weight. Fat will continue to be stored in the body until we help detox the liver. But the liver detoxes excess estrogen, too. So if you support the liver, this will reduce excess estrogen. This also means fat loss since estrogen is the hormone that holds fat in the cells.

Bile Is Important

The liver secretes bile, a fluid stored in the gallbladder, for release when needed for digestion. Bile is necessary for the digestion of fats and also assists in the absorption of fat-soluble vitamins A, D, E, F, and K, and helps assimilate calcium. A deficiency of bile can hinder fat digestion and slow proper bowel elimination.

Have You Irritated Your Gallbladder?

The gallbladder and liver are partners in "grime." Usually, if one is toxic, so is the other. According to Dr. Matsen,

> Gallbladder problems start when the liver is so overloaded with intestinal toxins that they get dumped into the duodenum or gall-bladder before they are fully neutralized. These toxins, if left in the

gallbladder can cause irritation. If the gallbladder doesn't secrete bile properly, the fats and minerals in the bile can become stones. The most common symptom of gallstones is feeling worse after eating fatty foods.[2]

If you eat a typical high-fat American diet, the overworked liver produces too much cholesterol, which crystallizes into gallstones. If your liver is too toxic, it may not produce enough bile to dissolve the cholesterol. But if you don't get enough fat in your diet, the cholesterol in the unused gallbladder can solidify and also create gallstones or high cholesterol! A common symptom of bile trouble is burping after meals or feeling pain between the shoulder blades.

Dr. Jonathan Wright in his book, *Dr. Wright's Guide to Healing With Nutrition,* states that gallbladder attacks could be completely avoided by eliminating allergenic foods from the diet. Dr. Wright reports that he hasn't had to refer anyone for gallbladder surgery since 1979. He must be on to something![3]

Doctor, How's My Liver?

Many of my overweight clients who have come to see me have blood test results from their doctors. According to their tests (SGOT, SGPT, alkaline phosphatase or bilirubin tests), there was absolutely no liver dysfunction. These standard medical tests look for liver enzymes in the blood and they are vital for spotting liver trouble if the liver cells are ruptured. However, according to Dr. Matsen, these tests don't pick up early-stage liver overload.[4]

A routine symptom survey that I run in my office shows that many people have an overloaded, sluggish liver. In fact Dr. Matsen believes that even people without the obvious symptoms may have an overloaded liver (fatigue, mood swings, PMS, irritability, and water retention). So if you are overweight, I recommend a liver support. Following my eating plan described in chapter 19 will support your liver to detox and help you lose fat.

Why Are We Toxic?

The average American consumes almost three pounds of food additives a year! Imagine that! There are over ten thousand additives allowed by the FDA that include MSG, harmful red and yellow dyes, BHA, BHT, and artificial sweeteners that few of us can spell or pronounce. Many fruits and vegetables are waxed to retain moisture, but the waxes are toxic.[5]

The air we breathe is contaminated, and our fast-food American diet of high-fat, sugar, and salt does not give our bodies enough nutrients to maintain proper health. What happens to these chemicals and toxins in our body? They overload the eliminative organs, especially the liver. The result is that most Americans are fatigued or tired. Toxic people always feel tired!

A toxic body is also an overly acidic body, which is not healthy. According to Harvey and Marilyn Diamond in their book, *Fit for Life,* a toxic system is characterized by bloating, excess weight, cellulite, graying hair, balding, nervous outbursts, dark circles under the eyes, and premature lines in the face.[6]

What Hurts the Liver?

Many of the foods that we grew up eating hinder the liver's functioning. As my client, Jill said, "These are foods we were encouraged to eat. But our parents didn't intentionally set out to hurt our digestive systems. They didn't know the effect of processed foods on our liver."

THE WORST OFFENDERS

- Drinking caffeinated beverages and/or alcohol

- Smoking cigarettes

- Eating fried foods and saturated fats

- Eating foods made from white flour

- Eating foods that contain white sugar

- Eating a diet high in red meat

- Overeating

- Eating large meals late at night

Smoking and Your Liver

We all know smoking is unhealthy. As you become healthier, it will be easier to quit smoking. I suspect smoking helps people gain weight since the nicotine adds to the toxicity of the liver. While smoking does not aid your ability to lose weight, most people can still lose weight even if they smoke. They may need the following nutritional support: flaxseed oil, B complex, antioxidants, and a liver and colon detox.

High-Fat Foods Are Dangerous

Dr. John McDougall's book, *The McDougall Plan,* states that a diet of rich, high-fat, low-fiber foods is the cause for the following diseases:

DISEASES COMMON AMONG PEOPLE OF AFFLUENT SOCIETIES		
Medical Conditions	**Bowel Disorders**	**Cancers**
Atherosclerosis	Chronic diarrhea	Breast
Heart attacks	Constipation	Colon
Strokes	Hemorrhoids	Prostate
High blood pressure	Appendicitis	Ovary
Obesity	Diverticulitis	Kidney
Adult-onset diabetes	Diverticulosis	Body of uterus
Gout	Crohn's disease	Testicle
Uric acid kidney stones	Ulcerative colitis	Pancreas
Calcium kidney stones	Malabsorption	Lymphoma
Osteoporosis		
Multiple Sclerosis		
Psoriasis		
Gallbladder disease		
Tooth decay		
Acne and oily skin		
Food allergies[7]		

What Can I Do?

The eating plan described in chapter 19 is designed to cleanse your liver and assist you with safe weight loss. Cleansing or detoxing the liver is vital for weight loss. This means eliminating stimulants and toxic foods. But there are other steps you can take to support your liver.

In an article that appeared in *Total Health* Magazine, my friend and nutritionist Willa Vae Bowles writes that lemon is the most valuable food for the liver. It's the only known food that contains diluted hydrochloric (HCl) acid for protein digestion. (HCl was discussed in detail in chapter 3.)

Fresh lemon can be converted by the liver into more different enzymes easier than any other natural substance. She recommends putting the juice of a lemon in your drinking water throughout the day. Or first thing in the morning, have the juice of a lemon in warm water sweetened with honey, molasses, or the herb, Stevia. (See chapter 12.)

Bowles further states that lemons can help regenerate the liver, purify the glands and cells, increase energy, dissolve toxins and mucus in the body, and restore HCl to the stomach.[8]

It's a wonderful food to add to your salad dressings. Lemon will help the stomach, the liver, and will aid fat-burning efforts! Here is a classic cleansing drink that has helped many people through the years:

Lemon Drink

> 8 ounces pure water
> juice of ¹/₂ lemon
> Optional: 1 teaspoon honey, Sucanat or dash of Stevia
> (See chapter 12.)

One of the best things you can do to support your liver is get plenty of exercise and eat a clean, healthy diet high in vegetable protein and low in refined, processed foods and saturated fats.

Juicing for the Liver

Drinking vegetable juices for two to three days really helps the liver. Here's a recipe that I give my clients:

> 6-8 carrots
> ¹/₄ beet
> 1 apple
> 1 stalk celery

Juice this combination and drink once a day, preferably in the morning. If you have low-blood sugar or you are insulin resistant, juicing isn't recommended. (See chapters 8, 12–13.) With your doctor's permission, you might want to consider following a juice fast for one or two days. See Cheri Calbom's book, *Juicing for Life* in the Bibliography.

Liver/Gallbladder Cleanse

The liver and gallbladder cleanse is often recommended for cleansing these organs. However, I highly recommend that you do this under the supervision of a health care professional.

I've counseled people who have tried to do a liver/gallbladder cleanse at home, not realizing the importance of first cleansing the colon. Some have gone through unnecessary pain as the body attempted to eliminate gallstones into a clogged colon.

Your health food store carries several types of liver support including Milk Thistle X and Liva-Tox by Enzymatic Therapy, and Milk Thistle extract by Solary. Common lipotropics are Lipotropic Metabolizer by

---

WHAT ELSE CAN I DO?

In addition to drinking the lemon water daily, here are more tips to support liver health:

- Eat a diet of 50 percent raw fruits and vegetables

- Lipotropics are compounds that help promote improved liver function and fat metabolism. Formulas contain choline, methionine and inositol.

- Take a B complex supplement daily.

- Take a liver support herb called Milk Thistle, 200 mg., three times a day. (Milk Thistle, also called Silymarin, helps enhance bile production and liver function.) Dandelion root and parsley are wonderful for the liver, too.

- Take one tablespoon of flaxseed oil daily

- Take antioxidant supplements (vitamins A, C, E and the mineral selenium)

- Take a garlic supplement—two capsules, three times daily.

Country Life, Lipotropics by Nature's Life, and Lipotropic Plus by Kal. I use Livaplex, Hepatrophin PMG, AF Betafood, Cholacol or Choline by Standard Process.

How and When Are You Eating?

Your liver can only process so much food at one time. It's much better to eat small meals. Habitual overeating is hard on your liver. Eating late at night is also hard, because that's when your liver wants to rest.

WHAT SHOULD I AVOID?

Additionally, some foods just aren't good for the liver:

- Avoid pork and shellfish.

- Avoid red meats and dairy products until the liver is well.

- Avoid most saturated fatty and fried foods, including trans fats.

- Avoid processed, refined starches, and white sugar.

Are You Retaining Water?

Many women over thirty retain water. A sluggish liver is almost always related to water retention in the kidneys. There are many causes of water retention, among them: liver or kidney dysfunction, hormonal imbalances, allergies, excess sugar and carbohydrate intake, and salt.

The most obvious place to start is to limit salt consumption to less than 2,000 mg. a day. This requires a lot of label reading, but as you will see, most natural foods are low in salt. Processed and refined foods, on the other hand, are high in salt. (For sodium tips, see Appendix C.)

A supplement that would help is a natural B^6, three times a day. Take B^6 along with a natural B complex.

Drink more water, not less. Most people who guzzle sodas all day are depleting their bodies of potassium. Replace the soda with water or with juices made from raw fruits, which are high in potassium. A 90 mg. potassium supplement may help with water retention.

About Alcohol

Tissues in the liver can be repaired even after years of abuse. However, alcohol does damage to the liver that may never be repaired. Alcohol overtaxes the liver, causes dehydration and causes vitamin and mineral deficiencies. For good health, long life and weight loss, I recommend you avoid all alcohol.

Nutritional Summary

- Drink the Lemon Drink
- Take digestive enzymes
- Juice carrots, beets, and apples daily
- Take a B complex supplement daily
- Take liver support herb such as Milk Thistle
- Take one tablespoon flaxseed oil daily
- Take a lipotropic
- Take antioxidant supplements (vitamins A, C, E and the mineral selenium)
- Take a garlic supplement—two capsules three times daily

What I eat matters. I now choose to eat the right portions that are right for me. I eat when I'm hungry and stop when I'm full. I no longer want to overeat. I love how good I feel when I support my liver.

PART THREE

What About Thermogenics and My Thyroid?

For I will restore health unto thee.
Jeremiah 30:17

Chapter Six

Are You Revved Up or Burned Out?

Have you ever seen an advertisement nailed to a stake at a busy intersection that reads:

> *Lose Weight! Feel great without suffering! Eat the foods you love and still lose weight! You don't even have to exercise!*

Yeah, right, and Elvis is still alive, too!

Unsafe Fat Burning

This ad is for thermogenics or nutrients that increase the metabolic rate and suppress the appetite. Certain foods and spices such as cayenne pepper, ginger, mustard, and cinnamon increase your metabolism and are safe. The right kind of exercise also increases thermogenesis.

However, some stimulants can raise insulin and actually hinder fat burning, so it's important to make a distinction between safe and unsafe thermogenic agents. A brochure for one of these supplements instructed the consumer to: *minimize foods high in fat; minimize foods high in sugar, consume moderate amounts of carbohydrates, increase dietary fiber and water.*

If the consumer followed these instructions, he or she may have no need for a thermogenic supplement! The problem is, in searching for a quick fix, people try the thermogenics *before* they try to cut back on fats, exercise regularly, and eat a balanced diet. These lifestyle changes may be all that was needed to lose weight. Instead they saw thermogenics as the only choice; it is not.

Lose More Than Weight

Earlier I mentioned empty promises of some weight loss products. I've seen dozens of products sold on street corners and in shopping malls. Unfortunately, these products are often inferior, high priced, and scary. Sure, people may "lose weight quickly" but since this goes against how our bodies are designed, it also means good health can be lost just as quickly!

Is this how you buy your groceries, an electrical appliance, or fine clothes? Why purchase something as important as a nutritional supplement from someone you have never met, who probably has little knowledge of nutrition, from a company that may be encouraging such sales gimmicks?

Additionally, many of these sales people never ask about your heart, thyroid, or if you are pregnant or diabetic—concerns that are found on all of these supplement labels.

Health Alert

Herbs like ma huang/ephedra, guarana, yerba mate, kola nitida, kola nut, and bissysnut contain caffeine which is an artificial stimulant. They give you a buzz that will indeed cause a degree of fat-burning. Be aware, however, there are dangers associated with high caffeine intake. These herbs tend to *overstimulate and even wear down your adrenals,* eventually causing fatigue. The biggest danger is that these supplements never get to the root cause of the problem such as poor digestion or unbalanced sugar levels. In nearly every case, people gain all the weight back again, because they never changed their diet nor did they deal with the health conditions that may have caused the weight gain in the first place.

How Are These People?

Have you ever met someone who lost weight and kept it off on these products? Is their health okay? Do they now have heart or adrenal problems? I frequently consult people who suffer from the terrible side effects.

Some time ago one of my clients named Debbie, dragged herself to my office suffering from chronic fatigue. She had taken such products for three years. The high caffeine caused her body to become nutritionally deficient and her immune system to be impaired. No one told her it wasn't safe. They told her it was "natural."

She decided to stop using it "cold turkey," and ended up on the couch for three weeks. Her energy levels were so low she could hardly function. She needed diet coke and chocolate in order to gain enough energy to get off the couch! She went from being ten pounds overweight, to being fifty pounds overweight!

I put Debbie on nutritional support for adrenals. In the beginning she could barely work for three hours at a time. A few months later, she was able to handle a full day's work, and she's progressively getting better and better.

Pay Day's Coming!

If you insist on taking these products, realize that sooner or later, you will have to deal with the consequences of burned-out adrenal glands, which may take months to restore!

People tend to apply the rule "if a little is good, more is better," to weight-loss supplements. However, that's not true with these herbs. Caffeine and herbal stimulants especially, should not be taken in excess! They are powerful stimulants and caution is needed.

A Further Word of Caution

People with high blood pressure, thyroid imbalances, heart irregularities, women with fibrocystic breast disease, and pregnant or lactating women *should not use* ephedra or products that contain ephedrine. Always consult your physician before taking these products if you are taking any prescription drugs.

And if you have been taking these products, you'll have to wean yourself off of them slowly. You'll need nutritional support. I highly advise you to see a nutrition-minded health professional.

Your Mighty Thyroid

Your body's metabolism depends on your thyroid. The thyroid produces the hormone thyroxine. If too much thyroxine is secreted, it causes high-thyroid function (hyperthyroidism). If not enough thyroxine is secreted, it causes low-thyroid function (hypothyroidism), which can lead to obesity. The most common symptoms in low-thyroid function are:

COMMON SYMPTOMS OF LOW-THYROID

- Fatigue
- Cold hands and feet
- Brittle nails
- Pale skin
- Ringing in the ears
- Reduced initiative, depression

- Weight gain
- Dry, lifeless hair; thinning hair
- Mood swings
- Constipation, gas, bloating
- Menstrual irregularities, PMS

Herbalist Louise Tenney says the glands need to be functioning properly in order to ensure harmony among the body functions.[1] If one gland is not healthy, others will be thrown out of balance to make up for the deficiency. If the hormones are imbalanced, it is harder to lose weight.

How's Your Thyroid?

Over the past several years, people have come to my office because of a weight problem, stating that their thyroid is perfect. "My blood test said my thyroid was okay," they tell me.

For years, this bothered me. In some cases, it was obvious that the person's thyroid function was impaired, so why didn't it show up in the blood test? I finally learned a good explanation from Dr. Cass Ingram. He says,

> However, be aware that these [blood] tests are often normal even if the thyroid gland is malfunctioning. That is because the tests show only how much thyroid hormone is circulating in the blood and tell nothing of how well the hormones are functioning on a cellular level. Additionally, the loss of up to 70% of thyroid function may occur before blood tests become abnormal. The fact is thousands of Americans have thyroid glands which are operating at 10 to 30% capacity. No wonder so many individuals suffer from chronic fatigue.[2]

The late Dr. Broda O. Barnes, a world renowned thyroid authority, discovered the relationship between body temperature and the thyroid. Here is a simple test developed by Dr. Barnes that you use to determine if your thyroid is underactive:

THE BARNES BASAL TEMPERATURE TEST

1. Shake down thermometer and place it by your bed before retiring.

2. Upon awakening, before getting up, take your temperature under your arm and hold thermometer for fifteen minutes without moving.

3. Record the temperature and date.

4. Do this for three to five days in a row.

Your basal body temperature should be between 97.6° and 98.2°F. Anything lower can indicate hypothyroidism and anything higher could indicate hyperthyroidism (hypothyroidism can mean weight gain).[3]

What Hurts Your Thyroid?

Poor diet (malnutrition) and lack of exercise are the main causes of low thyroid. Eating foods that hinder the thyroid function make you gain weight! Processed foods are toxic to the body. They also hinder your body from working properly—especially your precious thyroid. Here's a short list of the worst contenders:

CONTRIBUTING FACTORS TO LOW THYROID

• Coffee	• Lack of exercise	• Sugar
• Alcohol	• Cookies	• White flour
• Cake	• Excess estrogen	• Candy
• Ice cream		

Healthy Foods Can Harm Too!

However, according to Dr. Ingram, certain otherwise *healthy* foods may also be harmful to the thyroid function. These include: raw soybeans, cabbage, broccoli, rutabaga, cauliflower, kale, Brussels sprouts, watercress and peanuts. If you eat these foods, he recommends that you cook them in order to inactivate the interfering chemical known as a goitrogen.[4]

What Can I Do?

If you are hypothyroid, (low thyroid) how can you assure that your thyroid gland will function normally so you can lose weight? Something you can do is add more iodine-containing foods to your diet such as saltwater fish (halibut, cod, herring, and haddock), and take food supplements like kelp and essential oils (such as flaxseed oil). Kelp tablets, sold at health food stores are excellent sources of iodine. You need only a small amount of iodine (50-150 mcg). Have your nutritionist check your levels of zinc and selenium. A B-complex supplement is important, too. The amino acid L'tyrosine can boost the thyroid.

But before taking an isolated amino acid, get your amino acids from foods like eggs, chicken, and so on, or take an animo acid supplement which contains *all* of the amino acids. Then add isolated amino acids. Taking 500 mg. of L'tyrosine in the morning can help you eliminate the need for a morning caffeine fix. *However, be very cautious about taking this or any other isolated amino acid supplement. First, check with your doctor if you are taking any medications at all, since combining amino acid supplements with medications may cause unwanted side effects.* Only plan on taking these supplements for one to three months. Remember, most low thyroid problems stem from poor nutrition. If there is no change after taking this or other supplements, see your doctor.

You can find desiccated thyroid at your health food store, too. I use Organic Iodine and/or Thyrotrophin PMG by Standard Process. Enzymatic Therapy makes a product called Thyroid and L'Tyrosine Complex, but you can find separate L'tyrosine from several other companies.

See a health professional who can write a prescription for a natural thyroid hormone supplement. He or she may additionally recommend various herbs or homeopathic remedies for better thyroid function.

For the name of an M.D. or D.O. who is familiar with the Barnes test and natural solutions to thyroid problems, call the Broda Barnes M.D. Research Foundation at (203) 261-2101.

Eat Fat to Burn Fat

Scientist Brian Scott Peskin, author of *Beyond the Zone,* says: "Increasing the amount of the body's brown fat and minimizing intake of carbohydrates (even natural ones) are the only natural ways to increase the body's metabolism."[5] How can you increase your body's brown fat? Peskin's scientific answer is to take essential oils. (See chapter 14 for more about these oils.)

To burn more fat, we need to eat more fat, and limit refined sugar and carbohydrate consumption because all excess carbohydrates are converted to fat.

How About a Chocolate Shake!

Clients are always asking me about weight loss supplements that boost the body's ability to burn fat naturally. Through the past twenty years, I've looked at dozens of products, many of which have come and gone! I've even tried some. I can remember one particular product that seemed to be effective as long as I no longer wanted to sleep for the rest of my life! Not a good trade-off in my opinion.

About Other Shakes

Products such as Slimfast or even Ensure are no more than low-fat, high-sugar junk food. The Center for Science in the Public Interest (CSPI) called Ensure "a useless baby formula for seniors—a mixture of sugar, oil, water and protein plus vitamins and minerals."[6]

Slimfast is a popular drink that works because it's a liquid diet. However, it contains sugar and hydrogenated oils. You can achieve some results drinking these liquids, but you will probably gain all the weight back. Look for a balanced protein or meal supplement powder from a health food store. Here are some recommendations: Fulfill by Nature's Secret, Nature's Plus Spiru-tein, Natureade Vegetarian Protein, Super Green Pro by Nature's Life, and Twin Lab Veggie Fuel. Designer Protein by Next Nutrition is a good ion-exchange whey base protein. All weight-loss supplements will be more effective when accompanied by a healthy whole-foods diet, eliminating foods that depress the thyroid such as white bread, white flour, and white sugar.

Nutritional Summary

- See a health professional about a natural thyroid hormone
- Take a kelp or natural iodine supplement
- Check your zinc and selenium
- Take a L'tyrosine supplement
- Take desiccated thyroid supplement
- Take the B complex

I get the energy I need from good healthy foods, and not from dangerous pills. My body burns fat perfectly. I eat the right foods to support my thyroid.

PART FOUR

Why Am I
So Tired?
The Usual
Suspects

I will praise thee; for I am
fearfully and wonderfully made.
Psalm 139:14

Chapter Seven

Are You Sneezy, Grumpy, and Dopey?

"Yeah, I'm gonna start an exercise program. Really, I can't wait. I know what I'll do. I've even bought a new outfit with matching aerobic shoes. It's just that I'm so tired! I think I'll take a nap instead. Maybe later..." You know what happens next? Nothing!

When Trisha came in to see me, she had an enzyme deficiency, a sluggish thyroid and liver, slow adrenals, low iron, and chronic fatigue. I asked her if she were doing any type of exercise, and she assured me she was not.

Are You Too Tired to Exercise?

Throughout the years, one of the most common complaints I hear from clients is: "I'm too tired!" And since I experienced years of lethargic, couch-potato fatigue, I believe them! Trisha's health issues had to be addressed first. After her energy levels came up, *then* she felt like exercising.

As a personal fitness trainer, I am a firm believer in regular exercise. (See chapter 17.) But some clients need nutritional support in order to have energy to exercise. I recommended nutritional supplements for Trisha:

- Antioxidant vitamins (Vitamins A, C, E, and selenium)
- B complex
- Multiple vitamin/mineral supplements
- Help for her thyroid and adrenals
- Iron
- Digestive enzymes

What Makes Us Tired?

When clients come into me with complaints of low energy, and since there are many reasons for lack of energy, I've become an energy detective. Here's what I've found.

POSSIBLE ENERGY ROBBERS

- Excess carbohydrates sugars, or coffee (processed foods again!)
- Sluggish thyroid
- Sluggish adrenals
- Sluggish liver
- Hypoglycemia (low-blood sugar)
- Allergies
- Candida Albicans
- B vitamin deficiency
- Iron deficiency
- Zinc deficiency

See Your Doctor

The adrenal and thyroid glands are energy-producing glands, and your health care professional can help you if this is the root of your fatigue. He or she can also check your vitamin and mineral levels for possible deficiencies.

What About Fibromyalgia?

Besides chronic fatigue, another common problem is fibromyalgia. I have several clients diagnosed with fibromyalgia who became pain-free in four months after changing their diets and taking whole-food nutritional supplements. An excellent book on this subject is *Reversing Fibromyalgia* by Joe M. Elrod.

Cleanse Your Bloodstream

Most of my clients can't believe how great they feel following a cleanse like the one I mentioned in chapter 4. As discussed earlier, excess toxins zap your energy reserves. These toxins are everywhere—in the air we breathe, (the only place you can see them is in Los Angeles!) in the water we drink, and in the food we eat. Our bodies store these toxins. This hinders the natural fat-burning process. These toxins also make you tired. So that's the first area to consider when you are dragging around listlessly. I highly recommend starting with a simple colon/bloodstream cleanse to help eliminate fatigue.

Secondly, I check for allergies, which we will look at in this chapter. In chapter 8, we'll look at low-blood sugar, and in chapter 9 we'll talk about Candida Albicans.

Ah-Ah-Ah-Choo! Those Allergies!

When I was in my twenties, I had a continual runny nose. No matter what I tried, the symptoms would not leave. Most of the time, I felt like a combination of Snow White's friends: Sneezy, Grumpy, Sleepy, and Dopey! Mine was not an isolated case. In the United States, about forty million people suffer from some type of allergy.

As I began to study nutrition and health, I learned about food allergies and discovered that I was allergic to milk. When I stopped drinking milk, my runny nose problem left completely and has never returned! More importantly, however, my body stopped retaining water, and weight loss became easier.

Where Are They Hiding?

More and more people are discovering that hidden food allergies cause many different uncomfortable symptoms, including weight gain and fatigue. If you experience any of these symptoms, you may have food allergies:

COMMON SYMPTOMS OF FOOD ALLERGIES

• Sneezing	• Sniffling
• Headaches	• Dry throat
• Aches	• Coughing
• Irritability	• Skin rashes
• Gas and bloating	• Depression and mood swings
• Rapid pulse after eating	• Hot flashes
• Constipation or diarrhea	• Severe cravings or addictions
• Dark circles beneath the eyes	

How Much Healthier Can You Get?

I remember in the 1970s, I made whole-wheat pancakes from flour I had personally ground just an hour before. The pancakes were terrific. After eating them, I promptly fell asleep. I didn't know this at the time, but falling asleep after meals is a common symptom of allergies — especially to wheat products.

Cravings and Weight Loss

Food sensitivities can cause people to crave the foods to which they are allergic. When I was a compulsive overeater, I continued to crave and eat these allergens, such as wheat products. I didn't realize that my cravings were based on allergies. When I tried to eliminate these foods, the withdrawal symptoms caused irritability, and I was never satisfied.

Sugar Again

In her book, *Lick the Sugar Habit,* Dr. Nancy Appleton gives additional insight into allergies. The foods people are generally allergic to, such as milk, corn, wheat and chocolate are almost always eaten with sugar. Appleton suggests that it's this sugar combination that causes them to become allergens. She further points out that most Americans have grown up eating eggs with a glass of orange juice. The sugar from the orange juice, exhausts the enzymes needed to digest the eggs. The answer? Drink the orange juice before eating your eggs, giving your body enough time to digest the juice.[1]

Dr. Ingram goes a step further saying that sugar depletes the immune system. That's why sugar sensitivity and allergies are common. He believes that when people have sugar allergies, it shows poor adrenal gland function because a high-sugar diet stresses the adrenal glands.[2]

The stuffy nose and watery eyes that plagued Dr. Appleton while she was growing up, she now knows were signals of undigested protein.[3]

Instead of seeing these reactions as symptoms of a disease, it's better to see them as signals from the body that something is out of balance.

ADD/ADHD

Allergies are commonly involved when children or adults have the symptoms of ADD or ADHD. Certified Nutritionist Marcia Zimmerman has written an excellent book using a thirty-day diet and nutritional plan that I highly recommend for anyone with these conditions. Additionally, Dr. Mary Ann Block's book devotes an entire chapter to allergies and their relationship to ADHD. Both books are listed in the Bibliography section.

Allergies and Added Pounds

Why is it important to know if you have allergies? Food allergies irritate sensitive body tissue; the inflammation causes the body to retain fluid—and you know what that means! Weight gain.

Allergens can also depress the thyroid gland, and a sluggish thyroid gland means weight loss is slow. Also, foods that trigger allergic reactions can set off binging. Once you are addicted to a certain allergen, you eat compulsively to keep feeling good and avoid the discomfort of withdrawal. You can become addicted to any food—even healthy foods—that you eat or drink daily, and usually we are not aware of these addictions.

But Isn't it Healthy?

Yes, even "healthy" foods (especially whole-wheat bread) can be addictive and be an allergen. If you've ever tried to withdraw from one of these foods, you know what I mean. When you stop eating them, it's uncomfortable because they are addictive. We've eaten them because we craved them and without them we go nuts. The truth is, we have to go without them "for a season" in order for the allergic symptoms to leave.

Start With the Stomach

Dr. Matsen writes that allergies can be caused by foods that are not digested properly. If foods are not broken up completely during digestion, then very small particles of undigested protein are still in the blood. These molecules are treated by the bloodstream's immune system as foreign invaders. They provoke an antibody response trying to eliminate these invaders. Matsen states that if people will rebuild the digestive system, they will slowly detoxify and desensitize the body to where individual foods are no longer a problem.[4]

COMMON ALLERGENS

• Shellfish	• Wheat	• Corn
• Soybeans	• White sugar	• Milk
• Eggs	• Chocolate	• Coffee
• Caffeine	• Peanuts	• Citrus fruits
• Additives	• Yeast	• Beef
• Pork	• Eggplant	• Tomatoes
• Mushrooms	• White potatoes	• Tobacco
• Red and green peppers	• Cayenne	• Paprika

How do we know what foods we are allergic to? A good place to start would be with your family doctor who can administer tests for determining allergies. Below is also a test you can do at home that will help you to pinpoint some allergens.

Simple, Quick Allergy Test

Take a six-second pulse rate and multiply by ten to get your resting pulse rate. It's normally between 52-70 beats per minute. Eat the foods that you are testing for an allergic reaction. Wait 15-20 minutes and take your pulse again. If your pulse rate increase more than 10 beats per minute, omit this food from your diet for a month and retest.[5]

Drugs taken to treat allergies simply mask the symptoms. They do suppress the allergy symptoms, but they also hinder the effectiveness of the immune system.

What Can I Do?

If you suspect food allergies, then:

1. Replace oranges with mildly acidic fruits like kiwi fruit and strawberries.
2. Ditch the gluten. Replace wheat products with oatmeal, including oat flour, millet, barley and brown rice.
3. Try rye bread, oatmeal bread, buckwheat bread, millet bread, and barley breads in place of whole-wheat bread.
4. Take a cultured acidophilus tablet daily or eat acidophilus yogurt daily—you know, the good stuff, not the cappuccino or aspartame-sweetened stuff!

5. Don't drink your milk! Replace it with soy milk, rice milk, or use homemade applesauce in cooking or on cereals.
6. Make your own salad dressings with olive oil and lemon juice or apple cider vinegar.
7. Improve your digestion by taking lemon water in the morning.
8. Eat grains like wheat, rye or oats in the sprouted form, which makes them more digestible.
9. Eat many raw, fresh fruits and vegetables.
10. Work on better elimination and liver health, following the suggestions in this book.
11. Handle sugar cravings by supplementing your diet with Chromium GTF or L'glutamine. (Also see chapter 8 on low-blood sugar, chapter 9 on Candida and chapter 10 on cravings.)

What Does it Look Like?

Here is a sample of a non-allergenic meal plan.
Breakfast: 2 eggs with a slice of soy bread OR soy protein smoothie drink OR ½ cup oatmeal with apple juice or soy milk
Lunch: A green salad with chicken strips and lemon/olive oil dressing, vegetable soup, and millet bread
Dinner: Grilled salmon with steamed vegetables and a side salad

What Else Can I Do?

If you are serious about ridding your body of allergens, I recommend that you eliminate *all* milk and dairy products and even whole-wheat products for a month. If many of your symptoms leave, you can suspect you have allergies to milk or wheat.

What else can be done to win this war over allergies? Here are a few more suggestions that will help your body to handle all foods better:

- Build up the digestive system with digestive enzymes and follow the principles of food combining.
- Help the adrenal glands by eliminating stimulants like coffee and sugar.
- Build the immune system by eliminating all refined sugar and supplementing the diet with the antioxidant vitamins (A,C, E, and selenium), garlic, and essential fatty acids.

- Take an amino acid support.
- Eliminate all diet drinks.

We've only skimmed the surface regarding food allergies. An excellent book is *Allergies: Disease in Disguise*, by Carolee Bateson-Koch, D.C. For further reading, see the books on allergies listed in the Bibliography. Also, see the Resources in Appendix J.

Nutritional Summary

- Eliminate possible food allergens
- Take digestive enzymes
- Eliminate stimulants like coffee, sugar, and all diet drinks.
- Supplement the diet with the antioxidant vitamins (A,C, E, and selenium), garlic, and essential fatty acids
- Supplement your diet with Chromium GTF or L'glutamine if you are struggling with starch, sugar or alcohol cravings

I no longer have to drag myself around. I can eat foods that give me energy. I know which foods make me tired and it's easy to eliminate them or substitute healthy foods.

Chapter Eight

Sugar-High Got You Low?

W hen I was a compulsive overeater, my favorite binge foods were sugars and carbohydrates. The only problem with my sugar-high was that it always made me blue.

The Sugar Cycle

When we eat too many simple or refined sugars such as cookies, candy, and doughnuts, the pancreas reacts by producing too much insulin and the result is a drop in blood sugar. Insulin is called the "hunger" hormone, but it's also the fat-storing hormone. Eating sugar-full foods causes you to get on the never-ending cycle of:

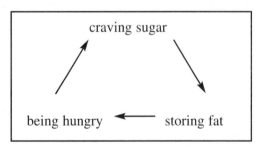

In order to lose weight permanently, we have to handle hunger and sugar cravings.

Do You Have Low-Blood Sugar?

The condition I had was low-blood sugar (hypoglycemia). Generally, the normal blood sugar range is between 80-120 mg. of glucose. Abnormal blood-sugar levels are considered anything above 160 or below 65. Below 65 indicates low-blood sugar, and there are thousands of people walking around with these symptoms.

**SYMPTOMS OF
LOW-BLOOD SUGAR**

Fatigue	Cravings
Heart problems	Depression
Dizziness	Headaches
Irritability if meals are missed	

A diet high in sugar can cause continual cravings, increased appetite, and weight gain! Excess food and especially excess carbohydrates or sugars turn to fat in the liver. If we support the liver and handle the sugar imbalance, it's easier to lose fat.

Burn Fat or Store Fat—It's Your Choice!

The two hormones that are secreted by the pancreas are insulin or glucagon. You want to eliminate insulin-producing foods and add glucagon-producing foods. The chart below shows what foods stimulate what hormones.

FAT-STORING FOODS AND BEVERAGES STIMULATE INSULIN PRODUCTION

Candy	Cookies
Cake	Ice Cream
Pretzels	Corn chips
Potato chips	Bagels
Refined white bread	Refined white pasta
Most sugared beverages	High-starch vegetables (corn, carrots, potatoes)
Coffee, Tea	Sodas

FAT-BURNING FOODS AND BEVERAGES STIMULATE GLUCAGON PRODUCTION

Fish	Lean Meat
Turkey	Eggs
Tofu	Tempeh
Soy burgers	Soy milk
Cottage cheese	Whole-grain breads
Most fruits	Low starch vegetables
Oatmeal	Rye bread/crackers

I'm Always Hungry!

Your pancreas secretes insulin in response to high-starch, high-sugar, and high-fat foods. For many people, eating sugar and carbohydrates doesn't cause weight loss but rather weight gain, cravings, and hunger. Additionally, you can have a high insulin response by:

1. Overeating. Just eating too much food can cause greater insulin response.
2. Eating too many carbohydrates at one meal—simple or complex; healthy ones or processed ones, it doesn't matter.
3. Not eating enough protein or fat at a meal or in one day.
4. Eating too much protein or fat at a meal or in one day.

I'm Burning Fat!

When insulin is high, glucagon is low and vice-versa. So if you want to burn fat instead of store it, you need to eat less carbohydrates and more protein. Adding protein to meals stimulates the release of glucagon, which helps your muscles burn fat. Protein also helps build muscle mass. Don't be afraid of eating good quality protein and good fat.

What Happened?

Most of us who grew up eating processed cereals, white bread and processed snacks have "stressed" our pancreas. We were originally designed to be able to eat *some* healthy carbohydrates. However, our stressed pancreas can't handle high amounts of carbohydrates.

A quote in the current best-selling book, *Sugar Busters* (written by four medical doctors) puts the sugar story into perspective: "The pancreas gland was probably not called upon to secrete as much insulin in *one day* of an *entire lifetime* as it is called upon to secrete nearly *every day* of a modern postinfant lifetime."[1]

Young children and teens are showing up in my office not only with weight problems but also with serious blood sugar imbalances, including Type II Diabetes and ADD/ADHD. The epidemic size of these imbalances was unheard of one hundred years ago, when the average American only ate twelve pounds of sugar, compared with the national average of 160 pounds of sugar per person, per year. I am so concerned about the children of this nation! Parents around the country feed their little ones sugar as though it were a healthy food. It's not! (See chapter 12 for details and the Bibliography for books on sugar, allergies and ADD.)

Eating Disorders

Why wouldn't eating disorders such as anorexia or bulimia be common among young women if their diets consist of sugar, sodas, and fried foods (devoid of vital nutrition)? It's as though our fast food industry sets them up for bulimia and anorexia. Most people with eating disorders are first, malnourished, especially in important minerals.

A zinc test that I routinely do in my office reveals that they are completely deficient in zinc, which is the mineral that helps us have a normal, healthy appetite. There is great hope for people with eating disorders, but the nutritional treatment must be aggressive and include the following: digestive enzymes, chelated zinc, antioxidants, amino acids, flaxseed oil, multiple minerals and vitamins. Eliminating non-nutritious substances like sugar, white flour and soda is vital.

(Parts Seven and Eight in this book will help you plan a lifestyle of healthy eating.) I highly recommend you work with a health professional, counselor, and invest the time and money it takes to help these people become healthy and whole.

The Glycemic Index

The Glycemic Index rates foods by how quickly they are converted to glucose, the form of sugar found in your blood. The lower the rating, the better they are for sustained sugar levels in your blood. (See the Glycemic Index in Appendix D.)

Using the Glycemic Index, choose most of your foods from the Low to Medium range. Eliminate refined, processed foods since these are generally higher on the Glycemic Index. However, just because it may be slightly higher doesn't mean you can *never* eat it. Our goal is to eat more whole foods in their natural state—these foods will be naturally lower on the Glycemic Index. If you eat higher glycemic foods with protein and fat, they are less likely to be stored as fat than if you ate them alone.

Not Just for Diabetics

The Glycemic Index is vital to a diabetic, but applies to anyone who is trying to lose weight and has failed with the low-fat, high-carbohydrate diet. Here's why—the higher the glycemic factor, the more likely that food will be turned to fat in the body. And the more sugar or fat in a product, the more likely it will have a higher glycemic factor. Not surprisingly, the lowest glycemic foods are whole, natural, unprocessed foods like whole grains, beans, and vegetables.

To understand why certain foods can help with weight loss, it's good to look at a diabetic's diet, which includes cereal grains, legumes, and root vegetables. Simple sugars are restricted. Fiber is the key ingredient in this diet because it helps control blood sugar levels.

Beans Are Good for Diabetics

Beans are a vegetable and even fall in the category of a complex carbohydrate, yet they are a protein with a lower glycemic index. That's why beans, and especially soybeans, are so good for diabetics.

In their book, *The Simple Soybean and Your Health*, co-authors Mark and Virginia Messina report the connection between fiber and diabetes.

> The same fiber that helps to lower cholesterol levels also plays a role in regulating glucose levels. Soluble fiber—the kind found in oats, legumes, fruits, and vegetables—forms a spongy gel in the intestines. This gel slows the release of food into the bloodstream.[2]

A slow rise of blood sugar is easier to handle, and scientists have shown that this type of diet actually improves insulin sensitivity. What this means is that adding fiber makes it easier for diabetics to control their blood-sugar levels.

Not God's Idea

God made food to naturally help you maintain weight. He didn't make starchy foods without fiber. Man removed the fiber when he refined foods. When whole wheat is refined into white flour, it acts as a sugar and is stored as fat!

A good rule of thumb is the more processed the food, the higher the glycemic index. When you eat carbohydrates, eat those that are high in fiber and low in sugar. For example, fruit juices have a higher glycemic index than fruits, and white bread has a higher glycemic index than whole-wheat bread.

What Can I Do?

If you lack energy and suspect that you have hypoglycemia:

1. Have your doctor run a Glucose Tolerance Test.
2. Eat regular, small meals (3-6 per day).
3. Eat foods lower in sugar. Eliminate high-sugar foods, refined processed foods like instant rice and potatoes, pasta, white flour, sodas and alcohol.
4. Eat whole-grain cereals and breads, beans and lentils. You need some complex carbohydrates, but stick with those that are lower in sugar and higher in fiber. If you feel like taking a nap after a meal, you probably ate too much sugar or too many carbohydrates at that meal.
5. Eat a balanced diet and get enough protein, both animal and vegetable based.
6. Have some type of good fat. (See chapter 14).

It's not worth the brief moment of pleasure experienced when you eat too much or the wrong types of sugar, because your sugar high will cause the sugar blues. As you make the decision to eliminate sugar, don't think about giving up something. Instead consider how great you will feel, and all the wonderful health benefits you will gain.

Remember if you are hypoglycemic, it's best to stay off all sweeteners—anything that ends with "ose" such as lactose and glucose. (See chapter 12 for healthy sweeteners.)

What Can I Take?

1. Chromium is essential for normal blood sugar levels. Most Americans are low in chromium, possibly due to the high intake of processed, refined white sugar that contributes to a chromium deficiency. Take 200 mcg. daily. I have successfully used a Standard Process product with my clients called Cataplex GTF, which is chromium GTF or Glucose Tolerance Factor. Your health food store will carry a local brand like Natures Plus Chromium GTF or New Chapter GTF Chromium. Some of my clients have used chromium picolinate, another type of chromium, which doesn't seem to be as effective as chromium GTF.

2. Take the antioxidant vitamins A, C, E and selenium.

3. Take a B complex supplement. Dr. Bruce West in his article in "Disease and Prevention" says that thousands of people with hypoglycemia are really suffering from a B Complex deficiency called B Complex Deficiency Syndrome (BCDS).[3] Only pure, natural food-based supplements will overcome this deficiency. However, this supplement isn't as effective if you continue to overeat starches and sugars! Remember, the B complex vitamins are vital for carbohydrate metabolism. (I prefer using a Standard Process supplement called Cataplex B. Look for whole food, natural B complex supplements at your health food store.)

4. Additionally, eat a diet high in fiber emphasizing raw nuts, raw seeds and some beans. These foods are high fiber, which allow a slow release of insulin in the blood.

5. Most people who struggle with sugar, starch or alcohol cravings don't eat enough protein. First, make sure you get at least 20 grams of protein at each meal. If that doesn't help, try taking an amino acid supplement from your health food store. Finally, try taking a separate amino acid, L'glutamine, which energizes the body and can help eliminate sugar, starch or alcohol cravings. Take 500 milligrams in the morning or afternoon on an empty stomach.

There are many good books on sugar listed in the Bibliography. *Get the Sugar Out* by Ann Louis Gittleman, and *Lick the Sugar Habit* by Dr. Nancy Appleton are excellent. *Sugar Busters*, co-written by four authors, and *Sugar Blues* by William Dufty are also great. The *Stevia Story* by Donna Gates is a great book on how and why to use stevia.

> ### FOODS RICH IN B VITAMINS
>
> • Whole grains
>
> • Brewer's yeast
>
> • Raw nuts
>
> • Raw seeds
>
> • Green leafy vegetables
>
> • Fish
>
> • Organically grown eggs and
>   poultry

Nutritional Summary

- Take Chromium GTF (200 mcg.)
- Take antioxidants: A, C, E and selenium
- Take the B complex supplements (25-50 mg.)
- Eat a high-fiber diet
- Take L'glutamine supplement (500 mg. on an empty stomach, only with your doctor's permission)
- Eliminate high-sugar foods
- Exercise at least two to three times every week

Now that I know that refined white sugar stores fat, it's easy for me to give it up. I love the taste of natural sugar found in dried and fresh fruits. I love how good I feel when I eat right!

Chapter Nine

Is Candida Driving You Crazy?

Candida—sounds like a hot new car from Chevy, doesn't it? It's not a car, but it can drive you crazy!

What Is Candida?

Candida Albicans is a type of yeast that is naturally found in our bloodstream. Problems start when there is too much or an overgrowth of this yeast called *candidiasis* or *Candida Albicans.* Candida may also be the basis of allergies, depression, and various environmental sensitivities.

Yeast infections are epidemic and can turn even a sweet, loving person into a raving maniac. Imagine simultaneous itching, pain and burning. I'm health-minded and have rarely taken any pharmaceutical drugs for twenty years, but I was ready to take anything when I had a yeast infection several years ago. I thank God for my twin sister, Jackie, who waited on me hand and foot. By taking acidophilus and making some dietary changes, I survived.

Do You Have These Symptoms?

I've counseled women who live with the terrible symptoms of *Candida Albicans:* fatigue, colitis, constipation, heart burn, vaginitis, kidney and bladder infections, hyperactivity, hypothyroidism, and adrenal problems. Candida is definitely related to weight control and allergies. Dr. William Crook, in his book, *The Yeast Connection,* names fifty-five symptoms of this condition alone.[1]

I've met many women who suffer with a variety of these symptoms. They feel guilty because they can't stick to a diet, and have no energy to exercise. Well, who could with those symptoms? It's no wonder many women feel "out of touch" with their bodies.

How About You?

Dr. Lindsey Duncan says that over 90 percent of the US population has some type of Candida overgrowth. Here are some of the major symptoms listed from his Candida Self-Analysis Test.[2]

Use this gauge for each of the symptoms listed:	
No symptoms	**0**
Occasional or mild	**3**
Frequent and/or moderately severe	**6**
Severe and/or disabling	**9**

_____1. Constipation
_____2. Diarrhea
_____3. Bloating
_____4. Fatigue or lethargy
_____5. Feeling drained
_____6. Poor memory
_____7. Feeling "spacey"—hard to focus
_____8. Feeling moody or despaired
_____9. Numbness, burning or tingling
____10. Muscle aches
____11. Nasal congestion or discharge
____12. Pain and/or swelling in the joints
____13. Abdominal pain
____14. Spots in front of the eyes
____15. Erratic vision
____16. Cold hands and feet
____17. Women—Endometriosis
____18. Women—Menstrual irregularities and/or severe cramps
____19. Women—Premenstrual tension
____20. Women—vaginal discharge
____21. Women—persistent vaginal burning or itching
____22. Men—Prostatitis
____23. Men—Impotence
____24. Loss of sexual desire
____25. Low blood-sugar
____26. Anger or frustration
____27. Dry patchy skin

TOTAL _____

Add your total to determine your score. Use this breakdown to determine if your symptoms are yeast-connected.

Women:	
73	Almost certainly
49	Probably
24	Possibly
Less than 24	Probably not yeast connected
Men:	
56	Almost certainly
36	Probably
17	Possibly
Less than 17	Probably not yeast connected

Don't Kill the Good Guys, Too!

People most susceptible to Candida are ones who have taken antibiotics in the past. Antibiotics literally kill bad bacteria in the intestinal tract but they also kill the "good guys" (friendly bacteria). Other causes for Candida are eating refined sugars and the use of birth control pills.

Candida yeast grows on carbohydrates, preserved, processed and refined foods, molds, yeast, and gluten breads. Candida prefers starches and sugars, not proteins and fats.

Sugar Is Their Treat!

Since the yeast feeds on sugars, the best treatment is to stop eating sugar! Get off all sugars, even natural ones I already mentioned such as honey, maple syrup, and molasses. When I had a serious yeast infection, I was taking a night-time cold medicine, which was loaded with refined sugar. The sugar in the cold medicine kept feeding the yeast, and I had to eliminate all refined sugars, especially the cold medicine.

The one exception to this is the herb, Stevia (see pg. 130), which you can purchase at your local health food store or at the address at the end of this book. (See chapter 12.) Eliminate all junk foods and refined carbohydrates, too. Kiss your Twinkies goodbye along with ice cream, sweet rolls, cakes, cookies, pies, candy, and canned foods. No wonder you can lose weight on an anti-Candida diet!

ELIMINATE:

- Gluten bread and yeast baked goods
- Refined carbohydrates (pasta, white bread, bagels, pancakes, pastries)
- Dairy products (except for yogurt or kefir products)
- Dried, pickled, and smoked foods
- Mushrooms
- Nuts and nut butters (except almonds)
- Fruits, fruit juices and dried fruits
- Coffee
- Soda pop
- Black tea
- Caffeine
- Carbonated foods
- Alcohol, pickled, or cured foods
- Other yeast-related foods that you will want to watch are: aged cheeses, fermented foods such as soy sauce, tomato sauce, and candied fruits

---

What Can I Eat?

You may be thinking, *Gosh, Lorrie, so what can I eat then? Seaweed soup? Sweet and sour tofu?* The best diet to combat Candida is one with animal or vegetarian protein, and lots of vegetables. Hey, but that's not all! Eat simple, low-fat, low-sugar, foods like chicken and steamed vegetables.

HERE'S A GOOD FOOD LIST:

Onions	Garlic	Cabbage	Broccoli
Leaf lettuce	Poultry	Fish	Turkey
Lamb	Veal	Eggs	Olive oil
Butter	Seeds	Brown rice	Beans
Oatmeal	Quinoa	Millet	Tofu
Yogurt	Filtered water	Tempeh	Soy foods

By observing a strict diet regiment, Candida sufferers usually begin to experience improvement within one to three months.

More Help

1. Eliminate the yeast feasts. Avoid antibiotics, corticosteroid drugs, and birth control pills.
2. Cleanse dead yeasts and waste cells from body with a soluble fiber cleanser, which can be purchased at the health food store.
3. Strengthen your digestive system, especially the liver. I recommend a good all-purpose digestive enzyme formula, and that you follow the principles of good food combining. (See chapter 3.)
4. Promote friendly bacteria in the gastrointestinal tract by taking an acidophilus supplement.
5. Rebuild the immune system by taking a good multiple vitamin/mineral supplement with A, C, E and selenium and take the herb, echinacea. The best supplements are made from whole foods such as brown rice and organically grown herbs. Take garlic supplements. (Kyolic has a brand that is odor-free.)
6. Killing the yeast is important. Apparently, the yeast can burrow a hole in the intestinal wall and leave a hole through which undigested food can pass. (As if you needed to know this on top of everything else!)

You can find Nature's Secret Candistroy, Twin Lab Yeast Fighters, Yeast Team by Nature's Now, or Candida Formula by Enzymatic Therapy available at your local health food store. I use a three-part Candida program called Microbac by Physician's Choice. It's a chewable probiotic that can eliminate yeast in six to seven weeks. I also like the Standard Process products, Lact-Enz and Garlic.

Anyone with a serious yeast problem should work with a natural health care practitioner. I highly recommend Cheryl Townsley's book, *Candida Made Simple*, and Donna Gates' books, *The Body Ecology Diet*, and *The Stevia Story*, which are listed in the Bibliography.

Consider doing all of the following to eliminate *Candida Albicans*.

Nutritional Summary

- Take a yeast killer
- Take digestive enzymes
- Take yogurt or acidophilus supplements
- Take antioxidants
- Take a garlic supplement

Simple, healthy foods are the best. I love to eat vegetables and good quality protein. This way of eating is easy. I love how good I feel when my body works properly.

PART FIVE

How Can I Beat Cravings?

Be not desirous of his dainties,
for they are deceitful meat.
Proverbs 23:3

Chapter Ten

I'd Die for a Twinkie!

During the 1970s, I lived in West Germany for two-and-one-half years. While living there, I found it was easier to manage my weight. Compared to the United States, food was harder to get! There were no twenty-four-hour Quick Trips, or Git-N-Go stores. No twenty-four-hour grocery stores. In fact, many grocery stores closed early on Saturday and stayed closed all day Sunday! All-you-can-eat buffets had not caught on yet. In contrast, Americans are surrounded by food! It's everywhere. And the servings are so big! It would take me several days to finish off anything in a "big gulp" size.

Food Abounds

Having access to food does cause us to eat more, and even crave more. Overeating is definitely a detriment to good health, yet it's encouraged throughout our nation, and you can get food any time of day. On the surface, overeating seems harmless, but it can hurt your liver, your stomach, your health, and shorten your life span. In this chapter, we'll start with food hunger and then look at various food cravings.

Consider your body and how it functions. Do you have to do anything to keep your heart beating? No, it's automatic. If your body can control thousands of functions without your conscious help, why not allow it to tell you when to eat? It's unnatural to use appetite suppressants to override the body's signals. When you are hungry, your body is trying to talk to you. Once you begin to receive proper nutrition, you can trust your body's signals.

But I'm Always Hungry!

First, if you are hungry or thirsty all the time, see your doctor to rule out the possibility of diabetes or some other serious health condition. Second, take a close look at your diet. Are you eating a large amount of processed carbohydrates, such as breads, pasta, and other flour products? As I've already mentioned, eating refined, processed carbohydrates can make you feel hungry. Third, could a deficiency of fats be the reason you are so hungry? For example, in your desire to eat a low-fat diet, have you cut out all fat?

Unnatural hunger and cravings will disappear when your nutritional needs are satisfied with good fat. I know you've heard and read that all fat makes you fat. The truth is the right kind of fat will help you burn fat! (You'll find more details about this in chapter 14.)

Still Hungry?

If after adding good fats to your diet, you find that you are still having trouble with hunger and overeating, the following suggestions may help.

1. Take digestive enzymes with your meals. If you are not digesting your food properly, this leads to overeating and food cravings. (See chapter 3.)
2. Cleanse your colon following the guidelines suggested in chapter 4. If the colon is not functioning properly you are only absorbing a portion of what you eat.
3. Cleanse or support the liver by following the guidelines in chapter 5.

Beat Food Cravings

Any eating plan that doesn't address food cravings is bound to fail. The good news is many cravings are due to nutrient deficiencies. When you eat the right kinds of foods for your body, these cravings fall away. Many people are overweight simply because they have food cravings, so when the cravings are under control, the weight comes off. Let's take a closer look at a variety of cravings.

Can't Resist Sugar?

Emily came to me complaining of low self-esteem, coupled with marriage problems. It's extremely hard to have a healthy relationship and be full of faith and positive expectancy with chronic low-blood sugar! (How many marriages have broken up because of chemical imbalances?) She explained that ice cream was the only thing that helped her feel good.

However, eating ice cream set her up for further sugar cravings. Eating sugar also caused a release of serotonin and beta-endorphins, which made Emily feel high, reduced depression, and soothed emotional pain, but only temporarily. This vicious cycle prevented Emily from losing weight.

I advised Emily to eliminate all of the high-sugar and high-fat foods she craved. A better way to safely boost serotonin is by eating complex carbohydrates like bread and pasta. Tryptophan is an amino acid that also aids in the conversion of serotonin. It's found in protein foods like turkey, chicken, seeds and nuts. I prefer that my clients get their protein from food sources. However, a popular supplement that contains tryptophan, called 5HTP, can help people with sugar cravings. Take 50 mg., once or twice a day, especially before bed. It's widely available in most health food stores and has been beneficial for people who suffer from depression, migraines, fibromyalgia and weight gain. Again, check with your doctor and *do not take* if you are taking any medications. (An excellent book on the benefits and uses of 5HTP written by John Morgenthaler is listed in the Bibliography. Also see chocolate cravings in this chapter.)

Do You Have a Deficiency?

A craving for sweets may signal a protein deficiency or a chromium deficiency. If this is the case, try taking a protein supplement, or a chromium supplement. (Refer back to chapter 8 regarding chromium and the amino acid L'glutamine supplement.) Lack of fruits or starchy vegetables in the diet can also cause sugar cravings. Eat more whole squash, sweet potatoes, and apples. With these simple changes in diet, the craving for processed sweets will probably go away.

Sugar Is Addictive

Have you ever noticed that the more sugar you eat, the more sugar you crave? Sugar combined with starch (white flour) is even more addictive. When refined sugar in candy, cookies, and ice cream are eaten, they are converted to fat and end up on your waist, hips, and thighs.

Eating sugar causes your blood-sugar level to increase. The pancreas then releases insulin to lower your blood sugar. However, if too much insulin is secreted, too much sugar enters the bloodstream, leaving you feeling cranky, irritable and depressed. When you're tired and stressed, guess what you crave? More sugar! It's an endless merry-go-round.

Additionally, drinking coffee or alcohol or taking recreational drugs can set up a sugar-craving cycle that leads to sugar addiction.

As I've mentioned earlier in this book, sugar cravings may be a result of a low thyroid, allergies, low-blood sugar (hypoglycemia), or Candida. (See chapters 6, 7, 8, and 9 respectively for dietary changes and nutritional supplement suggestions.)

Carbohydrate Cravings

When you crave carbohydrates, such as breads and pastas, this may mean that you are eating too many carbohydrates. (Or that your pancreas is overworked.) Eating too many carbohydrates—even healthy whole food such as whole-wheat bread—causes you to want more carbohydrates.

When you experience these cravings, willpower alone will not help to suppress them. Sooner or later, you will give into your cravings. Instead, you can nip cravings in the bud by eliminating all processed carbohydrates, and then limiting quality (natural) carbohydrates to two or three servings a day.

One client, Jessica complained of feeling tired, cranky, and unfocused. She craved carbohydrates. Her Food Diary revealed that she frequently skipped breakfast, and later would drink a diet Coke and eat a doughnut. Typically she grabbed her lunch at a fast-food restaurant. Her only healthy meal of the day was at night—if she wasn't too tired to prepare it.

Jessica didn't eat enough protein. Her diet consisted of many types of processed carbohydrates such as bagels, pasta, granola, and potato chips. Eating all these carbohydrates, especially processed ones, continually set up a cycle of more cravings.

What Can I Do for Carbohydrate Cravings?

Many people with similar complaints simply don't eat enough protein foods. Again, in our efforts to watch the fat, we have often cut out too much protein. I recommended that Jessica have a small amount of protein at every meal, accompanied by a small amount of complex carbohydrates. I've discovered that low estrogen/progesterone can cause carbohydrate cravings, too. (See chapter 11.)

I also advised her to eat regular meals and eliminate all refined processed foods as much as possible. She needed to eat more fiber and to exercise regularly. Jessica felt more energetic, focused, and easy going by her second appointment.

Most of my clients have difficulty losing weight as long as they are in this carbohydrate-craving cycle because excess carbohydrates are stored as fat. (See chapter 13.)

Caffeine Cravings

The reason for these cravings could be a weak adrenal gland. People eat these foods and drink these beverages for quick energy, and to stimulate their weak and tired adrenals. (Wake up, you guys!) However, the more stimulants a person consumes, the more he or she needs to get that "quick fix."

Stimulants can be extremely harmful. Instead of stimulants, people with depleted adrenals need to build these glands with proper supplements. Start taking natural vitamins B and C. Your health food store carries supplements for the adrenal glands including licorice root and vitamin C or raw adrenal supplements. I like using Drenamin and Drenatrophin PMG by Standard Process.

What Can I Do for Salt Cravings?

In my office I routinely use a symptom survey. Craving salty snack foods such as popcorn, corn chips, potato chips and pretzels is often another indicator that you have weak adrenal glands. In addition to the suggestions above, see your health professional for a good adrenal support.

I've already mentioned how important the thyroid is for boosting energy and the supplement L'tyrosine. Change your diet first, then work with your doctor if you suspect low thyroid or low adrenals. (See chapters 6 and 16 on low thyroid and caffeine, respectively.)

Chocolate Cravings

Mary felt well adjusted; however, she daily craved chocolate. When she first came to see me, she was eating a pound a day of chocolate and was fifty pounds overweight. Mary loved chocolate and couldn't imagine life without it.

On a weekly basis, I meet women like Mary who are on a chocolate binge. Having had these cravings for years, some during their monthly cycle, they have learned to give in and accept them. Many authors, in fact, tout the benefits of chocolate during this time. However, in counseling women over the past ten years, I've never been successful in helping them lose weight and keep it off by continuing to eat chocolate regularly.

Giving into your monthly craving for chocolate is foolish. Why continue to set yourself up for depression, binges, and a higher risk of fibroid problems from the increase in caffeine? There are better answers!

A Better Way

Chocolate boosts the serotonin level. When you are down or depressed, (low serotonin level), you crave chocolate, sugar or starches. (By the way, serotonin levels seem to drop a few days before a woman's menstrual cycle. This explains the strong cravings for chocolate and sugar that most women experience monthly.) After eating chocolate, sugar, or starches, serotonin is released causing you to feel peaceful and calm. Your sleep is better; life seems wonderful. But that's only a temporary relief. The chocolate, sugar and starches cause a further downward spiral.

Prozac and Zoloft are prescription drugs that also boost serotonin. The good news: We don't have a Prozac deficiency. We can boost our serotonin levels naturally. The safest way of course is to eat a diet rich in healthy proteins, good fats and complex carbohydrates. And supplements such as 5HTP, considered by some to be a natural version of Prozac, have been very effective in treating people with depression. (See *5HTP: The Natural Alternative to Prozac* listed in the Bibliography.)

Eat Healthy Meals

I put Mary on the eating plan described in chapter 19 of this book. She continued to eat three meals a day with a little protein in each meal. She ate a complex carbohydrate following her dinner, usually before bedtime. This gave her body the added carbohydrates needed to produce serotonin. She also took a magnesium supplement (See below.). She slept well, and her cravings went away. She is now on her way to healthy weight loss.

What Can I Do for Chocolate Cravings?
1. Chocolate cravings may mean a deficiency in magnesium. Take a magnesium supplement of at least 300-500 mg. per day. I use Magnesium Lactate by Standard Process.

2. Eat regular meals.
3. Have a small amount of protein at each meal.
4. Have a complex carbohydrate (one serving of oatmeal or a baked potato) before bed.
5. One of the best chocolate substitutes I have found is Wonderslim, 99.7 percent caffeine-free cocoa, with no fat or sugar added. I've used it to make brownies that are great. You can eat the chocolate without the harmful side effects.

Another possible substitute is carob. While it doesn't taste exactly like chocolate, some of my clients have acquired a taste for it. A variety of carob products can be found at the health food store ranging from plain carob powder to carob cookies.

What Can I Do About Cravings for Crunchy Foods?

This craving may indicate a lack of fruits, vegetables, nuts, and seeds in the diet which satisfy the natural need to crunch. Rather than eating junk foods like processed potato or corn chips, try eating whole-rye flat bread, toasted pumpernickel, or whole-grain rye bread, which are lower on the glycemic index. (See the Glycemic Index in Appendix D.) Or try toasting one of the sprouted wheat breads such as Ezekiel bread or Manna Bread. (This can be purchased at the health food store.) These are so delicious they require no jelly, jam, or butter. Try toasted pockets of pita bread. Whole-grain rye crackers are also good and are available at both grocery and health food stores. Rye crackers spread with unprocessed nut butter have a great flavor!

What Can I Do About Cravings for Dairy Products?

These cravings may indicate a calcium deficiency. If you take an absorbable type of calcium supplement—such as calcium lactate—the cravings will probably go away. The trick is to get the right kind and amount. (This may require the assistance of a health practitioner.)

What Can I Do for Fat Cravings?

Cravings for fat in the form of chicken-fried steak, bacon, sausage, and mayonnaise may mean that you are not digesting fats properly, or it may indicate a lack of the right type of fats. Take a digestive enzyme with lipase for fat digestion, and herbs that support the liver such as milk thistle. And ditch those processed, hydrogenated fats! (See chapters 3, 5, and 14.)

What Can I Do for Protein Cravings?

When you crave protein, it usually means that you are not digesting protein properly, or you aren't getting enough protein. You need the digestive enzyme protease. (See chapter 3.)

What About Off-the-Wall Cravings?

What about the more unusual cravings such as pickles or other munchies? Hulda Regehr Clark addresses this area in her book, *The Cure for All Diseases,* giving possible explanations for the cravings.

Pickles. They supply vinegar and are often loved by persons with little acid in their stomachs or a lot of yeast (vinegar is a yeast inhibitor). Start drinking water with lemon juice or water with apple cider vinegar and honey.

Bacon. The fat soothes the stomach and slows down digestion. Switch to butter and cream with meals (but with moderation!)

Ice cream. Ice-cold food stimulates the thyroid, therefore, those people with low thyroid (hypothyroid) will crave ice cream. Follow the recommendations in chapter 6 for support for the thyroid.

Pretzels. You want salt plus the crunch. The answer for the need for crunchy foods can be found in foods such as apples, carrot sticks, raw nuts, and seeds.

Potato chips. You want salt, grease, starch and crunch. No wonder they are so popular! Again, the desire for crunchy foods can be satisfied with raw, natural foods.[1]

I have read dozens of books, many of which I would not recommend to my clients because they recommended eating the very foods with which my clients were struggling. Perhaps one of the best books written on this subject is the national best-selling book, *Potatoes Not Prozac* by Dr. Kathleen DesMaisons. Her entire book is designed to help you cooperate with the cause-and-effect relationship of brain chemicals and cravings.

Nutritional Summary

- Take digestive enzymes
- Cleanse your colon
- Support your liver
- Take a fiber drink
- Take a magnesium supplement for chocolate cravings
- Take the B vitamin complex
- Eat balanced meals
- For sugar cravings, suspect allergies, low-blood sugar, Candida, or low thyroid (See chapters 7, 8, 9 or 10, respectively.)
- Take a protein drink, or an amino acid supplement. Or consider taking 5HTP, L'glutamine, or L'tyrosine with your doctor's permission, since these amino acids should not be taken if you are taking any medications. Additionally, you should not take these isolated aminos at the same time. I would recommend the L'tyrosine in the morning, L'glutamine at lunch and the 5HTP at night. Your doctor can test your amino acid levels with a blood plasma test.

I only eat the foods I need when I am really hungry. I can and do resist junk foods. I'm breaking the craving/binge cycle. Cravings are a thing of the past because I eat balanced meals.

PART SIX

What Do Hormones Have to Do With Weight Loss?

Serve the Lord your God, and He shall bless thy bread, and water; and I will take sickness away from the midst of thee.
Exodus 23:25

Chapter Eleven

Are You Wacky for a Week?

Once a month the symptoms begin. Headaches, cravings, and "Please, just get me some chocolate!" We call it PMS, or pre-menstrual syndrome. Many husbands call it, "Punish My Spouse Syndrome."

When my clients tell me that they have tried everything to lose weight and they still can't, I suspect hormone imbalance. The thyroid gland is responsible for regulating your metabolic rate, or the rate that you burn calories. There is a strong relationship between the thyroid gland and hormones. Excess estrogen depresses the thyroid, but natural progesterone boosts the thyroid.

Do You Have Too Much Estrogen?

Dr. John Lee, author of the best-selling book, *What Your Doctor May Not Tell You About Menopause,* says that American women are estrogen dominant. This means they have too much estrogen and not enough progesterone. In American women, progesterone starts to decrease at about age thirty to thirty-five.

Estrogen, when unopposed or unbalanced by progesterone, causes estrogen dominance with undesirable side effects. This symptom commonly occurs in:

1. Estrogen replacement therapy
2. Premenopause
3. Exposure to xenoestrogens (fake estrogens)
4. Birth control pills (with excessive estrogen component)
5. Hysterectomy
6. Postmenopause (especially in overweight women)

Dr. Lee says:

> The key to hormone balance is the knowledge that when estrogen becomes the dominant hormone and progesterone is deficient, the estrogen becomes toxic to the body; thus progesterone has a balancing or mitigating effect on estrogen. There are very few Western women truly deficient in estrogen. Most become deficient in progesterone.[1]

Were You Raised in America?

If you were raised on dairy products (in America, who isn't?), then you have been bombarded with synthetic estrogens from hormones given to the animals we consume. Also, plastics and petroleum-based products in your normal household cleaners contain what is known as xenoestrogens or "fake" estrogens. These products are found in some soaps, pesticides, and perfumes made from petro chemicals. The molecule is so close to the estrogen molecule, that your body interprets it as estrogen. And if you already have a higher percentage of fat, then your body makes estrogen on its own. The hormone estrogen's job is to hold fat on us! So don't blame your hormone—it was just doing its job.

The Good News

According to Dr. Lee, a simple treatment with a natural progesterone can restore the balance between these two female hormones. Dr. Lee has been treating female patients with natural progesterone cream for the last 15 years. He says that the right amount of progesterone helps your body make natural estrogen. He points out a number of negative side effects caused by an imbalance of estrogen:

> Estrogen causes salt and water retention and high-blood pressure. Estrogen also opposes the action of the thyroid, promotes histamine release (which causes allergy-type symptoms), promotes blood clotting thus increasing the risk of stroke and embolism, thickens bile and promotes gallbladder disease, and causes copper retention and zinc loss. Estrogen unopposed by progesterone also decreases sex drive, increases the likelihood of fibrocystic breasts, uterine fibroids, uterine (endometrial) cancer, and breast cancer.[2]

What About Synthetic Estrogen?

One popular type of synthetic estrogen is derived from estrogen found in urine from pregnant mares. This synthetic estrogen is many times stronger than any woman's body would manufacture naturally. It is associated with a high risk of heart disease and several forms of cancer. Another popular combination contains synthetic estrogen and synthetic progestin. If you read the insert that comes with it, side effects include: blood clots, nausea, vomiting, breast tenderness, and abdominal pain. Yet it continues to be one of the top-selling drugs in the country.

Worse yet, taking synthetic estrogen depresses the thyroid, causing weight gain instead of weight loss. Most of my female clients who are on synthetic hormones say they gained weight in the hips and thighs after starting to take them.

Still other side effects of taking synthetic estrogen include: fibrocystic breast disease, cancer, and endometriosis. By the year 2000, cancer will be the number one cause of deaths in the United States, predominantly cancer of the breast and prostate.

In an interview, Cynthia Drasler a former pharmaceutical drug sales representative, stated,

> When I started selling chemotherapy in 1962, I was told that the breast cancer rate for women in this country was 1 in 14. When I quit the industry in 1990, the breast cancer rate for women in this country was 1 in 9. Now, I've been told that it is approaching 1 in 7. Obviously, something is very wrong with the way women are being treated in this country. When I read Dr. John Lee's book, I was amazed at the plethora of research he and others have done supporting the use of natural progesterone in the treatment of many women's problems both pre and post menopausally. I tracked down two of the studies that he cited and was very impressed with the high degree of statistical significance in them.[3]

One Woman's Struggle

Raquel Martin, author of *The Estrogen Alternative,* shares her experience struggling with menopausal symptoms.

> As I continued to ask questions, I began to understand that the doctors I had been seeing all along didn't necessarily have all the answers.

They didn't seem to comprehend completely the complexities of menopausal problems, the PMS problems of younger women, or the side effects of the synthetic hormones they were prescribing. Not only were their answers contradictory to each other; I sensed a lack of conviction on their part that this was indeed the right way to go. I thought to myself, *Is it any wonder women become confused, afraid, and discouraged during what can already be a stressful time!* [4]

Menopause Is Not a Disease

Chinese women have few, if any symptoms of menopause. Their high-soy protein diet is rich in phytoestrogens, a type of natural estrogen which has the benefits of synthetic estrogen without negative side effects. They don't even have a word for menopause in the Chinese language. Menopause is not a "disease" that has to be treated or cured. It is a natural process of life!

So Many Operations!

About 650,000 hysterectomies are performed in the United States every year, according to Dr. John Lee. And more significantly, most of the women treated for menopause still have symptoms and risks.

Not everyone even needs estrogen, often called Hormone Replacement Therapy (HRT). I have several clients who were not convinced they needed to take synthetic estrogen and experienced few if any menopausal symptoms.

Progesterone Helps Weight Loss

If we don't use synthetic estrogen and do use natural estrogen (such as soy products), what about progesterone? Instead of causing weight gain, natural progesterone helps weight loss. But there are other numerous benefits to natural progesterone.

Hormones, Cravings and PMS

Having a balance of natural estrogen and progesterone is vital for losing weight and curbing cravings. If estrogen levels are low, women often experience food cravings for fats, sugar or carbohydrates. Many of my clients have lost food cravings by using natural progesterone cream (which converts to estrogen in the body.) Additionally, here are some other natural solutions to hormonal and PMS symptoms and cravings:

For chocolate cravings, take 200 mg. of magnesium

For sugar cravings, use the progesterone cream, take Chromium GTF, or take the amino acid L'glutamine. (Take amino acid supplements only with your doctor's permission.)

For painful breasts, take an essential fatty acid supplement. (See chapter 14 on good fats.)

For painful periods, take 500-1,000 milligrams of calcium daily.

For depression, eliminate sugar and stimulants, increase your protein and consider taking 5HTP. (See chapter 10 on cravings.)

Cynthia Drasler told me in an interview: "I have been using a natural progesterone cream since February of 1997 with dramatic results. I had fibrocystic breast disease for twenty-two years. After three months of using this cream, my fibrocystic breast condition was gone. I was amazed and delighted. My only regret about natural progesterone is that I didn't know about it twenty years ago." [5]

Who Needs Natural Progesterone?

According to Dr. Lee, the woman who needs progesterone is any woman who:

- is taking estrogen replacement therapy
- is on the birth control pill
- has had a hysterectomy
- has been exposed to xenoestrogens
- suffers from PMS
- is trying to get pregnant
- has had a miscarriage
- has had breast or uterine fibroids or cysts
- is gaining weight in the hips and thighs
- is post or menopausal
- has a loss of interest in sex
- is depressed or fatigued
- is aging prematurely

Synthetic Progesterone

We have been discussing the benefits of natural progesterone. Synthetic progesterone (progestin) also has high risks associated with it:

birth defects, fluid retention, epilepsy, migraines, asthma, cardiac or kidney dysfunction, and depression.

Let's Compare

Below is a chart that compares estrogen and progesterone. The list is quoted from Raquel Martin's book *The Estrogen Alternative:*

CHARACTERISTICS OF ESTROGEN DOMINANCE	CHARACTERISTICS OF PROGESTERONE SUPPLEMENTATION
Weight gain	Utilizes fat for energy
Insomnia	Calming effect
Uterine cancer	Stops cells from multiplying
Fibrocystic breasts	Protects against fibrocysts in breast
Breast cancer risk	Helps prevent breast cancer
Depression	Natural antidepressant
Fluid retention (bloating)	Natural diuretic
Thyroid imbalance	Assists thyroid hormone action
Blood clots	Normalizes blood clotting mechanism
Migraine headaches	Restores oxygen to cells
Risk of miscarriage	Prevents miscarriages
Inflammation	Precursor to cortisone
Cramping	Relieves cramping
Elevated blood pressure	Regulates blood pressure
Acne	Aids in skin disorders
Irregular menstrual flow	Normalizes periods
Restrains bone mineral depletion	Stimulates bone mineral density[6]

Progesterone Cream

Since progesterone is very absorbable through the skin, the most common form of natural progesterone is a cream. Be sure to use a cream made from soybeans and yams (the whole potato yam so none of the nutrients are missing). Because it's a food product no prescription is needed for natural progesterone.

How do you know which progesterone cream to use? Read Dr. John Lee's book to help make the right choice. All wild yam creams are not the same. The cheaper the cream, the lower the percentage of natural progesterone. I carry a progesterone cream that we have sold to more than 2,000 women who tell us they love it. You can also find them in your local health food store.

If you are now taking HRT or some type of synthetic replacement, don't go off of it "cold turkey." You must wean yourself off of it. See a health-care professional who understands natural hormone therapy and alternatives to synthetic hormones. You can send for a kit to check your own hormone levels. (See Resources in Appendix J.)

How Do I Use It?

Dr. Lee recommends progesterone cream that is applied trans-dermally, which means "across the skin." The advantage is that it bypasses the liver and goes to specific receptor sites where progesterone is needed. Any excess is excreted from the body.

The general way to use progesterone cream is to apply ¼ teaspoon twice a day. If this is not enough to diminish hot flashes or PMS symptoms, increase to ½ teaspoon twice a day. A good cream lasts ten hours in the blood. Put the cream on the soft-tissue parts of your skin such as the inside of your wrists, inside your thighs, on your tummy, or on the underside of your arm (not where you put your deodorant!). Here are Dr. Lee's recommendations for using the cream.

1. Pre-menopause

If you are pre-menopausal or still menstruating, you only need the cream two weeks per month between day twelve to twenty-six of your menstrual cycle. Count your period as day one and count to day twelve. On day twelve, use the cream every morning and night for the next two weeks. If you experience cramps, rub the cream on your lower abdomen.

2. Those on Birth-Control Pills

Dr. Lee points out the numerous health problems caused by the birth control pill including depression, fluid retention, headaches, and liver disease. If you have been put on synthetic estrogen in the form of a birth-control pill, you could taper off the pill as shown in the following paragraphs and start using the natural progesterone cream. After you stop the pill, wait for your next period. Counting day one as first day of your cycle, count to day 12. Use the cream from day 12 to day 26 and then stop.

If your periods do not resume naturally after you stop the pill, use the cream every day except for 5 days in the month. When your period begins, stop using the cream. (Call your local library or bookstore for further information on natural birth control methods.)

3. Menopausal Symptoms (With Cycle)

If you have menopausal symptoms while still menstruating, use ¼ teaspoon twice a day, beginning with the eighth day from day one of menstruation until your next cycle.

4. Menopausal Symptoms (No Cycle)

If you have menopausal symptoms and are not menstruating, or you have osteoporosis, use the cream based on the calendar month. Use ¼ teaspoon on day 6 of each month and continue for the month until the last day of that month.

5. Those on HRT

If you are taking synthetic estrogen, you could reduce intake to a pill every other day instead of every day for the first two months. At the same time, take the cream according to directions as above. In the third month, cut your dose in half again or take one pill every four days while using the cream. Continue cutting dosage until you fully wean yourself off estrogen.

The easiest way to remember is take the cream, ¼ teaspoon morning and night, for three out of four weeks in the month, starting at the first week of the month. Then leave off for 5-7 days. A short period of no hormone cream increases estrogen receptor sensitivity.

6. Those on the Estrogen Patch

If you are using the synthetic estrogen patch, you could cut the patch in half and tape over the ends. Use it for one month, and then cut again (now in one fourth) the next month. Use the cream as previously instructed.

7. Those on Synthetic Progestin

If you are taking synthetic progestin, you can safely replace it with the cream. If you need extra estrogen, consider using Remifemin found at health food stores. Remifemin is a natural herbal estrogen product that has been used widely in Europe, Australia and the U.S. for menopausal symptoms.

8. Those on an Estrogen/Progesterone Compound

You could call your doctor and request just estrogen on a low dose. In six to eight weeks, cut in half. Then in another six to eight weeks take it every three days. If there are no side effects, it's all right to stop.

9. Those Who Are Thin

Most women can use progesterone cream without supplemental estrogen. The exception to this is women who go through menopause and are thin. (Since you are reading a weight-loss book, this is probably not you right now. But if you lose body fat and become thin during menopause, it does pertain to you.) Estrogen stays in body fat, so women who are very thin and have low-body fat do need an estrogen replacement, although not a synthetic one! If you have a question, have your hormone levels checked. Again, if you have a good percentage of body fat, your body will make estrogen, so you don't need supplemental estrogen.

Added Notes

If you start using the progesterone cream and you begin to bleed, there is generally no cause for alarm. What is happening is that excess estrogen is being eliminated. However, it's always a good idea to see your health care professional for any unusual bleeding.

Also, it should be noted that everyone is different. Some women need more cream than others. Try using one two-ounce jar a month for about three months, then cut back on the cream. If the symptoms return, resume your previous dose. But remember to stop using the cream at least 5-7 days every month to increase estrogen receptor sensitivity.

Bones and Hormones

Can progesterone help with osteoporosis? Yes! Natural progesterone also helps to thicken bone density.

Dr. Lee's research shows age to be no factor in this reversal of bone loss. One especially interesting response to natural progesterone cream therapy was with an eighty-two-year-old woman. After four years of using the cream, she had greater than 40 percent new bone density. Dr. Lee has proven that osteoporosis is not only preventable, but also reversible! A healthy diet and calcium supplementation is recommended. For an excellent hormone balance program, read Dr. John Lee's book.

A Healthy Lifestyle

Soy foods have been proven to help alleviate hot flashes. Soybeans are considered superfoods for menopause because they contain phytoestrogens, which are 1/400th of the strength of synthetic estrogens. Soy foods balance your natural hormone levels without any known side effects. Eating vegetable protein stimulates the liver to clear estrogens, increases progesterone and rids the body of excess estrogen. (See chapters 18-20.) A great soy cookbook is *Tofu Quick and Easy* by Louise Hagler.

Estrogen Dominance and Diet

We are eating too much food with estrogen. Remember, estrogen increases a woman's tendency to store fat. The typical American diet, high in process fats, sugars, caffeine and processed foods all increase the amount of estrogen in a woman's body. Xenoestrogens, which are estrogen-like molecules come from various types of plastics, pesticides and process fats. So eating at fast food places increases estrogen stores. We want to *decrease* estrogen and *increase* natural progesterone. Exercising regularly, taking natural progesterone cream and making the diet suggestions in this book will help you to decrease estrogen and assist your body's ability to burn fat.

FOODS THAT AGGRAVATE ESTROGEN DOMINANCE AND WEIGHT GAIN:

• Hydrogenated oils	• Red meat
• Coffee	• Alcohol
• Spicy foods	• Sugar
• Caffeine	• Artificial sweeteners

Add to your diet:

• Fiber	• Soy foods
• Calcium/magnesium	• Flax seed oil
• Evening primrose oil	• Organic iodine (for hot flashes)

A healthy nutrient-dense diet, with natural supplements will assist in both PMS and menopause symptoms. Be sure to refer to the Meal Planning and supplements in Part Eight.

Regular exercise is vital for good health, but also for relief from hot flashes, improved heart function, improved circulation, reduced blood pressure, improved ability to deal with stress, and increase in energy and endurance. Exercise also reduces risk of osteoporosis.

I highly recommend both Dr. Lee's book, *What Your Doctor May Not Tell You About Menopause*, and Raquel Martin's book, *The Estrogen Alternative*. Other excellent books are: *Super Nutrition for Menopause* by Ann Louise Gittleman, *Menopause Without Medicine* by Dr. Linda Ojeda, and *The Natural Estrogen Diet* by Dr. Lana Liew. An excellent soy cookbook is *Tofu Quick and Easy* by Louise Hagler.

All of these books are listed in the Bibliography.

Nutritional Summary

- Eat soy foods
- Take a calcium/magnesium supplement for painful periods.
- Take flaxseed oil or Evening primrose oil for painful breasts. (See chapter 10 about chocolate cravings; take 200 mg. of magnesium.)
- For sugar cravings, use the progesterone cream, take Chromium GTF, or take the amino acid L'glutamine. (Take amino acid supplements *only* with your doctor's permission.)
- For depression, eliminate sugar and stimulants, increase your protein and consider taking 5HTP. (See chapter 10 on cravings.)
- Use a natural progesterone cream

My hormones are balanced and my body works perfectly, as it was designed to work. I eat healthy foods to support my body. PMS, water retention, and cravings are gone. I am happy and healthy.

PART SEVEN

What Should
I Eat?

Why spend money on foodstuffs
that don't give you strength? Why pay
for groceries that don't do you any good?
Isaiah 55:2, TLB

Chapter Twelve

How Sweet Is Sugar?

Have you ever seen a Hershey bar tree or an M&M shrub? How about licorice on the vine? No! They are not "real" foods. Some of the ingredients in them may have originated from natural foodstuffs, but then they became processed. In chapters 12-16, we'll see what happens to these "non-foods" after we eat them.

Processed Foods Are Everywhere

Lisa Messinger, author of *Why Should I Eat Better?* tells us, "There is $400 billion floating around out there trying to get you to eat processed food, which is the largest industry in the United States. Food advertising is a $3.6 billion annual industry in this country, and almost a third of the ads include some type of health claim."[1]

**WHAT THE AVERAGE AMERICAN
EATS IN ONE YEAR:**

- 100 pounds of refined sugar
- 55 pounds of fats and oils
- 300 cans of soft drinks
- 200 sticks of gum
- 18 pounds of candy
- 5 pounds of potato chips
- 7 pounds of corn chips, popcorn, and pretzels
- 63 dozen doughnuts
- 50 pounds of cakes and cookies
- 20 gallons of ice cream[2]

What Are You Eating?

Several years ago, I was browsing through a fascinating book entitled, *4001 Food Facts and Chef's Secrets* by Dr. Myles Bader, when I came across these amazing statistics (that you just read on the previous page). These statistics are old. The current statistics say the average American eats 160 pounds of sugar per year! In the 1800s, individual consumption was about twelve pounds per year.

Dr. Bader says that during the last ten years, more than ten thousand new "convenience processed foods" have been introduced in the United States. What a staggering amount! On top of that, we spend billions of dollars on diets and drugs, yet in the world, our nation has some of the highest statistics of sickness and obesity.

Few Benefits

Most of the foods discussed in Part Seven earn the title of junk foods. Junk foods are not health-producing—not even "low-fat" junk food. They contribute to food addictions, heart disease, cancer, and diabetes. Remember that over-processed foods are not only void of essential nutrients and fiber, but they actually deplete the body of vitamins and minerals, causing nutrient deficiencies! They can truly be called "empty calories." Non-foods and artificial chemicals aren't harmless. They cause damage to your cells. Your body can't use them to make new healthy cells. What's even worse, these foods often irritate and upset our digestive tract. They have little nutrition, cost the body energy to process them, and they help you gain weight.

Processed foods could be hindering your weight-loss efforts, especially foods that you like so well and thought were so good for you but weren't! Where have those high-sugar, processed foods gotten you anyway? Better at fat storage.

No, Thank You!

When I was in my early 20s, I was the first one in line at the ladies fellowships to pile my plate full of sweets. I never thought I could give up sweets. Over the past twenty years, though, I could probably count on two hands the number of times I've eaten them. They just don't taste good anymore. Once you allow your body's natural taste to return, sweets may not taste good to you either. We *learned* to like them.

Is One Doughnut Harmless?

Let's compare a natural food, such as an apple, to a man-made food such as a doughnut. A doughnut contains white sugar, white flour, and hydrogenated fats. Because the doughnut contains few vitamins, minerals or enzymes, that empty food actually robs you of your store of vitamins, minerals and enzymes—the very nutrients you need to burn fat! This is the real problem.

Processed foods make a negative impact on you and your health. While we look at the doughnut as being harmless, it is the problem when it comes to nutritional deficiencies. In chapter 20, we'll walk you through a grocery store and show you how to select healthy, less-processed versions of these foods. In this chapter we'll talk about sugar, because it's the most prevalent and abused food in America.

What About Sugar?

I remember a conversation with some friends last year. They were counting fat grams so they could lose weight. In the same breath, they mentioned that they were going to fill up on diet coke and fat-free cookies! The message was clear: Fats were bad, but a little sugar is okay, and, in their minds, not even related to weight loss. Refined white sugar is one of the foods that causes your body to store fat. So it's not a healthy weight loss food! But is it healthy at all?

Sugar Was a Luxury

You and I may have grown up eating refined white sugar, but did you know that chemically refined white sugar is fairly recent? According to Mary June Parks in *A New You,* for centuries, sugar was sold by the tea-spoonful only through drug stores. Originally crude, unrefined beet sugar was a luxury. Sugar was served on rare occasions or used as a medicine for the treatment of gout.[3]

Our body was not designed to eat refined white sugar. When you eat it, you stress every digestive organ.

How Much Are You Eating?

Before we start, let's find out how much sugar you eat. Write down what you have eaten recently that may contain sugar.

_____

_____

_____

_____

_____

Sugar Is Fun, but it Makes Us Fat!

When we think of sugar, we think of fun, celebrations, and good times. Valentine's Day, Easter, Halloween, Thanksgiving, Christmas, birthdays and anniversaries all mean chocolate, candy, cakes, and sweets. We have all grown up associating good times with sugar treats. Individual consumption of sugar has skyrocketed, especially with the increase in low-fat or fat-free products. But over the past ten years, Americans have gained weight instead of lost weight! Why? When they took out the fat, they had to replace it with something—sugar!

Simple and Complex

Simple sugars like those found in fruit are good. But simple sugars that have been processed from fruits and even further refined are unhealthy. Complex sugars like those found in whole grains (barley or rice syrup) still contain vitamins, minerals, enzymes, and proteins if not processed over 130°F. In its natural form, sugar cane is a rich source of vitamins and minerals.

How Sugar Is Refined

Most people know that white sugar comes from sugar cane or sugar beets, but few know what happens in the refining process when they synthetically manufacture sugar.

It begins with a real plant food—sugar cane or sugar beets. Cane stalks are cut, crushed, washed, boiled, steamed, and then crystallized. Finally, it's filtered, cleaned and decolorized. Lime, acids and bleaching agents are added until it becomes the white, pure substance we recognize as sugar.[4]

The final product is so different from its original form that our bodies do not even recognize refined sugar as a food. It is no longer a true food—it's a synthetic substitute. No wonder it can give us a tummyache!

A Healthier Option

Refined white sugar is not your only option. That same sugar cane can be organically grown, and with minimal processing become a healthy sweetener commonly known as Sucanat. Sucanat retains natural color and trace minerals. (See the chart at the end of this chapter for healthy sugar substitutes.)

More Than Weight Gain

In her book, *Lick the Sugar Habit,* Dr. Appleton lists several health problems and their relation to white sugar: hypoglycemia, diabetes, constipation, stomach or intestinal gas, arthritis, asthma, headaches, psoriasis, cancer, osteoporosis, heart disease, obesity, Candida, tooth decay, multiple sclerosis, inflammatory bowel disease, canker sores, gallstones, and cystic fibrosis. She also cites several sugar "helpers": alcohol, caffeine (which can increase the amount of sugar in the bloodstream), drugs, rancid fats, overcooked foods, aspirin, food additives, and mercury.[5]

It's Too Much

Our pancreas was not designed to secrete as much insulin as is required by refined sugar. Constant insulin release results in the pancreas exhausting itself after years of refined sugar intake. Diabetes is caused by too little insulin produced and high-blood sugar levels. Eating refined white sugar immediately causes your blood-sugar level to rise and leads to a chromium deficiency. Fatigue is a common symptom of diabetes and hypoglycemia (low-blood sugar). Both conditions come from eating a diet high in refined sugars.

Out of Control!

In her book, *Menu and the Mind*, Mary June Parks discusses the relationship between a diet high in refined white sugar and violence. Right before their violent acts, the diets of these offenders included coffee, doughnuts, soda pop, French fries, white bread, and sugar. She quotes a study where certain prison inmates were not given junk foods with sugar, but rather were given vegetable proteins, whole grain breads and cereals, fresh fruits, vegetables, juices and some dairy products. Their diets were supplemented with B complex and vitamin C supplements. The simple alteration in diet plus supplementation resulted in excellent rehabilitation for most of those who participated in the experiment.[6]

Why Is There Violence in Our Schools?

Burgess Parks, Mary June's late husband, spent thirty-two years as a public school administrator. When he retired in 1970, there were only isolated cases of teachers being attacked. Today violence in schools is rampant. But no one is asking about their students' diets. She reports that when Dr. Schauss checked into the diets of juvenile delinquents, it was always sugar-laden junk food.[7] High amounts of sugar and soda burn up the B complex vitamins. Symptoms of a serious B vitamin deficiency are: anxiety, depression, mental confusion, insanity, irritability, and rage.

Want Better Teeth?

An interesting fact is that during World War II, some countries had to survive without refined, white sugar. Their incidence of dental disease and other illness dropped remarkably. Dr. Nancy Appleton says that until she stopped eating sugar, she had to visit the dentist every three months. Now that sugar is out of her diet, she only sees the dentist every six months, and even then, there is little or no plaque on the back of her teeth.[8]

Don't Keep Hurting Yourself

Additionally, sugar causes nutritional deficiencies, depleting your body of the B vitamins and many minerals. I like how nutritionist and author, Robert Crayhon, puts it:

> ...eating sugar is like hitting yourself in the head with a baseball bat. The less you do it, the better. Sugar always stresses the body. Healthy persons may not initially feel this stressing effect, but will eventually. By the time you feel it, it may be too late. Sugar may have claimed you as another victim of its subtle and destructive effects.[9]

Hidden Sugars Are Everywhere

You may be thinking, *I don't eat refined sugar—I'm safe.* You may not buy it intentionally, but it's everywhere! Of course you already knew sugar was in cookies, ice cream, candy, doughnuts, cakes, and pop. But were you aware that sugar is the number-one food additive hidden in many foods?:

FOODS THAT CONTAIN HIDDEN SUGARS

- Salad dressings
- Ketchup
- Mayonnaise
- Spaghetti sauce
- Peanut butter
- Soups
- Pickles
- Cereals
- Canned fruits
- Luncheon meats
- Vegetables
- Crackers
- Breads
- Pizza
- Juices

No one would intentionally sit down and eat several teaspoons of sugar at once. But they add up. Look at the number of teaspoons of sugar in some foods. Briefly look back to page 125. Can you add any more items to your list of foods that contain sugar?

AMOUNT OF SUGAR IN COMMON FOODS

Name of Food	Teaspoons of Sugar
1 ounce chocolate bar	5
12 ounces fruit drink	12
12 ounces cola	9
1/2 cup frozen sweetened fruit	6
1/2 cup fruit, canned in heavy syrup	4
1/2 cup fruit, canned in light syrup	2
8 ounces lowfat vanilla yogurt	4
8 ounces yogurt	7
1 cup ice cream	6
1 cup ice milk	6
1/8 of white layer cake with chocolate frosting	12
1/3 of 9" apple pie	12

Source: Adapted from "Dietary Guidelines for Americans," *Home and Garden* Bulletin No. 232-5, April 1986.

Read Labels Carefully

Refined sugar amounts to "empty calories." Labels are deceiving, so become "shopping detectives." Product ingredients are listed on the label in descending order by weight, from the greatest to the least. If a type of sugar is listed as one of the first three ingredients, or if there are several sugars listed, the product is high in sugar.

You may not recognize that a product has processed sugar in it because of its many different names: dextrose, maltose, honey, sucrose, sorbitol, lactose, glucose, and fructose. Here are others:

- Raw sugar
- Corn fructose
- Natural sugar
- Corn sweetener
- Yellow D sugar
- Corn syrup
- Cane sugar
- High fructose corn sweetener
- Brown sugar
- Caramel
- White sugar

I'm Safe—I Use Artificial Sweeteners

So you may have decided to switch to sugar substitutes. But wait. All things are not created Equal! Some actually leave you Sweet but Low. Let's look at two of the common ones.

Aspartame is two hundred times sweeter than sugar and has been used to take the place of saccharin in foods and drinks. Its major brand names are NutraSweet and Equal. It has been linked to PKU seizures, high blood pressure, headaches, insomnia, and mood swings. Several studies have shown immediate serious reactions to Aspartame: severe headaches, extreme dizziness, throat swelling, and other allergic effects, including retina deterioration. The worst thing is that none of these sweeteners satisfies our sweet tooth.

I Want More Food

Brian Scott Peskin reports that another problem with aspartame is that it pulls chromium from the body and actually triggers your appetite. One of Aspartame's components is methanol—wood alcohol! An excess of methanol can cause blindness or even death.

But Aspartame is everywhere—found in about five thousand products and it accounts for 80 percent of FDA food-related complaints. You'll see it added to ice cream, yogurt, fruit drinks, soft drinks, baked goods, and cereals.[10]

Saccharin is one of the common forms of sugar substitutes known as Sweet-N-Low, Sprinkle Sweet, Sugar Twin, and Sweet Ten. It comes from petroleum and is 300 times sweeter than sugar. Although the FDA proposed a ban on Saccharin after studies suggested a link between it and tumors in rats, it was saved by public demand for it and was left on the market. Its safety is under review.

They Don't Work!

Did you know that these sugar impostures not only can be damaging, but they can also make you fat? In the book, *The Body Signal Secret,* the authors Strauss and North quote an American Cancer Society study of 78,694 women, which showed that those who used artificial sweeteners were significantly more likely to gain weight than nonusers.[11]

Dr. Andrew Weil, author of *8 Weeks to Optimum Health,* says, "Avoid artificial sweeteners and foods made with them. They will not help you lose weight and are hazardous to your health." [12]

You don't need sugar substitutes! They upset your biochemical balance, hurt your health, and you don't need them to lose weight. As a shopping detective, notice the warning on the back of the Saccharin packet: "Use of this product may be hazardous to your health. This product contains saccharin, which has been determined to cause cancer in laboratory animals." Artificial sweeteners are made from coal-tar derivatives, which are indigestible. Many other countries have banned artificial sweeteners because of their link to cancer risk.

A Healthy Option

Wouldn't it be great if there was a sweetener with no calories, that inhibited tooth decay, was natural, safe for diabetics, and didn't feed yeast?

There is! Stevia is a small plant that grows in Latin America. It's been used for centuries by the Indians of Brazil and Paraguay to sweeten tea. The Japanese consume more stevia than any other country in the world, and Stevia now has wide commercial value in Japan to sweeten tooth-paste, soft drinks, chewing gum, frozen desserts, and other foods. It's two- to three-hundred times sweeter than sugar, yet it doesn't upset your blood sugar level. That's why it is successfully used by diabetics.

A whole food herb, Stevia helps prevent tooth decay and possibly can lower blood pressure, too. It helps control sugar cravings, and unlike sucrose and fructose, will not feed Candida yeast.

Stevia is available in the United States as a powder or liquid extract. Use one to two drops of Stevia to sweeten one cup of liquid. Stevia can be used for baking. Your health food store carries stevia made by: Body Ecology, Stevita, Wisdom of Ancients (black liquid extract), and Sweet Vibes (stevia with FOS). See the resource list in Appendix J for further information on how to buy Stevia.

What Can I Do?

1. Read labels. Realize that most of the processed foods available at the grocery store contain some type of processed sugar or corn syrup. Try to find products with little or no added sugar. See chapter 20 for a long list of healthy alternatives to your favorite sugar-sweetened foods.

2. Start to cut down on the number of foods that you are eating that contain sugar. Look for fruit-sweetened snacks. Don't keep sugar-sweetened snacks in the house.

3. Substitute for white sugar by following the chart at the end of this chapter. For example, instead of one cup of white sugar, use one cup of Sucanat.

4. Finally, don't buy refined white sugar and all synthetic sugars. Try Sucanat, brown rice syrup, barley malt, natural honey, blackstrap molasses or Stevia.

5. Take appropriate supplements (See chapter 8).

What Foods Contain Sugar?

How is it possible for one person to eat an average of 160 pounds of white sugar per year? Sugar is the number one food additive. Even Snack Wells products, touted to be "fat-free" are full of sugar. If our local grocery store aisles are full of highly processed, sugar-laden, high-fat foods, then we must be able to spot them and avoid them. I have compiled a list of common foods you will want to avoid or replace. You can purchase "healthy" versions of your favorite treats at your local health food store. Or, you can make some of these at home. Remember, excess sugars and starches cause weight gain. So move in the direction of eliminating them. After awhile, you may even find that you no longer need most of these foods!

FOODS TO ELIMINATE

Doughnuts	Commercial ice cream
Pastries	Candy bars
Cookies	Hard candies
Cakes	Sugar-sweetened cereals
Pies	Sugar-sweetened beverages
Brownies	Sugar-sweetened applesauce
Malts	Sugar-sweetened pudding
Sherbet	Salad dressings
Sodas	Barbecue sauce
Fudge	Whipping cream
Ketchup	Processed foods
Relish	Canned fruits and vegetables
Gelatin	Chewing gum
Jellies	Artificial sweeteners
Jams	Non-dairy creamers
Preserves	Cured luncheon meats
Marmalades	Graham crackers

Listed below are the names of healthy, natural alternatives to white sugar. They are available at your local health food store. I recommend Donna Gates' book, *Cooking With Stevia*, for help using stevia.

HEALTHY SUGAR SUBSTITUTIONS

For one cup of sugar, use:	Reduce liquid by:
Sucanat, 1 cup	1 cup
Fruitsource, $1/2$ cup	$1/4$ cup
Devan sweet (rice sugar)	$1/2$ cup
Honey, $1/2$ cup	$1/4$ cup
Molasses, $1/2$ cup	$1/4$ cup
Maple syrup, $1/2$ cup	$1/4$ cup
Date syrup, 1 cup	$1/4$ cup
Date sugar, 1 cup	$1/4$ cup
Barley malt, $1 1/4$ cups	$1/4$ cup
Fruit juice concentrate, $1 1/2$ cup	$1/4$ cup

It's easy for me to give up sugar. I love natural fruits and natural sweets. I have self-control. Sugar has no more power over me.

Chapter Thirteen

Can Pasta Make Me Fat?

Certainly, processed foods must have been around for a long time, but eating fast-foods and processed foods certainly wasn't God's idea from the beginning. I can't imagine Adam and Eve in the garden looking for Twinkies or Ding Dongs. Besides, we all know they much preferred apples!

The Grain, the Whole Grain, and Nothing But the Grain

There are three main parts of any whole grain: 1) the bran, which is the outer layer; 2) the germ or inside of the base of the grain; and 3) the endosperm or the starch in the center.

A whole grain refers to the entire grain—the bran, the germ, and the endosperm. Processing whole grains separates the bran and germ, which are necessary to digest the starch.

How Much Fiber Do We Need?

A good place to begin to understand the impact of processing of food is with whole grains. Most Americans eat between seven to ten grams of fiber per day; a safe range is between twenty-five and thirty. People in some third-world countries who experience much lower rates of disease eat almost four times more fiber than we do—forty, sixty, and even one hundred grams per day.

Lack of fiber is one of the primary preventable causes of colon cancer! And Americans spend more than $600 million a year on laxatives. Cancer, heart disease, arthritis were not even common until after the refining of white flour.

Traditional Foods are Often Health Foods

Complex carbohydrates have always been valuable in traditional, long-lived cultures, and today science confirms that a high-fiber diet contributes to preventing several cancers, including colon cancer. We may lower our chances of developing cancer by eating more beans, brown rice, and seeds. Prostrate, colon, and breast cancer are high in cultures that eat a diet high in red meats and lower in cultures that eat beans, seeds, and rice.

Are Bagels Fattening?

We've already discussed the Glycemic Index in chapter 8. Let's review why we should eat whole grains and not processed ones. White flour is pure starch without the B complex and vitamin E. Refined white flour is "fattening" for at least two reasons.

1. Eating white flour products causes the pancreas to secrete insulin, and insulin is the fat-storing hormone. So you probably will have difficulty losing weight until you pass up those refined carbohydrates: white flour, white cakes, white cookies, white pasta, and so on.

2. Up to 80 percent of the essential nutrients are lost in the production of white flour. After white flour is rolled, it's then bleached by chlorine dioxide where any vitamin E is completely destroyed. In the refinement process, more than 21 nutrients are taken out, and only a handful are put back in. White flour lacks the vitamins to help digest it. The bran and germ hold most of the vitamins and minerals in wheat. They contain the B complex, and trace minerals like zinc, copper and iodine. These minerals and the B complex are required for proper carbohydrate metabolism. In other words, you need these vitamins and minerals to properly process carbohydrates.

   Additionally, wheat germ is a great source of vitamin E, an important nutrient for heart health that is also an antioxidant, one of our best protectors against heart disease.

White, "refined and enriched" carbohydrates are a rip off. We can purchase wheat germ and wheat bran to supplement our diets, but it's better to eat the whole grain. Let's look at the different types of carbohydrates.

SIMPLE CARBOHYDRATES

- *Healthy*, simple carbohydrates found naturally in fruits are easily digested and assimilated.

- *Unhealthy*, simple carbohydrates that include processed foods, such as refined candy, cookies and cakes, are also quickly absorbed and converted into glucose. However, the result is a burst of energy that leaves as quick as it comes because these foods lack vitamins, minerals, and fiber.

COMPLEX CARBOHYDRATES

- High-fiber complex carbohydrates include whole grains and whole-grain products (bread and pasta) such as wheat, brown rice, oats, and barley.

- Lentils and beans such as pinto, red beans, black beans, and vegetables such as potatoes, carrots and onions are all healthy complex carbohydrates.

For many years, I have taught cooking classes on how to cook with whole grains and how to bake whole-grain bread. I have tremendous respect for these whole foods. I don't recommend a *high*-carbohydrate diet, but I do recommend eating several complex carbohydrates daily. (See chapter 18.) Don't cut out *all* starches—just limit your intake. Balance is the key here. *Some* natural complex carbohydrates are good. The problem is eating a meal or snack that is too high in carbohydrates. Combinations such as a bagel and coffee, cereal and juice, and pasta with vegetables are high-glycemic. So add protein to your meals and snacks and choose low-glycemic starches. (See the Glycemic Index in the back of this book.) Eliminate the processed, man-made carbohydrates—white bread, potato chips, corn chips, candy, cake, cookies, and so on.

What Can I Do?

1. Read labels. If the label says "enriched," it's not a whole grain. Look for the words "whole-wheat flour," and don't buy products with caramel coloring, which may be used to make the bread look brown. To test, squeeze the bread! If it's not firm, it's not whole grain!

2. Start to cut down on the number of foods that you are eating that contain white flour. Try not to keep white flour products in the house.

   Look at making these changes as a new adventure. Some of these foods may be new to you, but once you get started, you'll love it. One of my clients said, "Most people don't know that healthy food really tastes better. They don't realize that whole-grain breads are delicious."

3. Substitute whole-grain flours such as wheat, rye, or brown rice for white flour. Shop at bagel shops and bakeries that carry whole-grain bagels, muffins and breads, (nine-grain or oat bran taste great) or go to a health food store. French, sour dough and Italian breads are mostly white flour.

   Look for "sprouted" grain breads. They are so yummy! I used to bake these breads before they became commercially available. Grain (usually wheat) is sprouted, crushed, formed into a loaf and baked an hour or longer at very low temperatures. It's so sweet, it doesn't even need jelly or jam. These loaves are sometimes called Manna bread.

Purchase whole-grain breakfast cereals. (A more complete list is found in chapter 20.) Here is a short list:

Grape Nuts	Wheaties	Total
Shredded Wheat	All Bran	
100% Bran	Wheetena	
Ralston Cream of Rye	Old Fashioned Oats	

4. Finally, stop buying white flour products.

EASY WAYS TO GET MORE FIBER

1. Eat "five a day." Make salads, or buy already made salads at the grocery store.

2. Eat high-fiber cereals with two grams of fiber per ounce.

3. Add three or four servings of beans or legumes to your weekly menus. Add beans to rice dishes, salads, or pasta dishes.

4. Add other whole grain products like oats, millet or barley to your soups, salads, casseroles or main dishes.

5. Substitute whole grain flours like wheat or rice for white flour in recipes and add oat flour, or oat bran to baked goods.

6. Use pureed vegetables or beans to soups for additional fiber, texture, and creaminess.

7. Eat whole or dried fruit instead of drinking fruit juices.

8. Substitute whole-grain brown rice for white rice.

What Foods Contain White Flour?

This next list is very long. But remember it is possible to find almost all of these products made with whole grains. See chapter 20 for healthier alternatives to these foods.

**FOODS TO ELIMINATE
(MADE WITH WHITE FLOUR)**

White bread	Commercial cereals
White hamburger/hot dog buns	Muffins
Corn bread	Doughnuts
White rolls	Sweet rolls
Croutons	Croissants
Dumplings	Fruit pies
Cookies	Batter breads
Pizza	Pita breads
Pastas and noodles	Most sweetened snack
Waffles and pancakes	foods
French toast	Creamed canned soups
Crepes	Breaded foods
Bagels	Pretzels
Corn chips (processed, then fried)	Saltines and crackers
Pot pies	

I love the taste of natural, whole grains and whole grain products. Refined snacks don't even taste good to me anymore. I love how good I feel eating healthy foods!

Chapter Fourteen

Does Fat-Free Mean Fat Loss?

W hen I ask my clients about the amount of fats they consume, the majority proudly announce that they don't eat much fat and their Food Diaries confirm this. Then I ask them how they like it—the majority announce to me that they don't like it and they miss their fat. What happens? They manage to squeeze French Fries and ice cream into their fat-free diet!

We're Born With a Fat Tooth

God made us with a desire to eat and enjoy fat! I've tried no-fat diets, and you probably have, too. After a few days, you go nuts looking for the most fatty foods you can find! I remember looking for oil for my salads, or butter for my bread! Going no-fat is no fun!

I was so pleased to learn that these desires are not unnatural cravings that we have to suppress, fix, or eliminate, but rather our natural, normal, healthy, God-given desires for an important nutrient—fat! In this chapter, we'll explore various fats. But let's look at fat-free foods and their role in weight loss.

Do Fat-Free Products Work?

The key to weight loss is to work with the body, not to try to fool it with partial, processed, made-up foods like low-fat substitutes. After working with hundreds of clients, here's what I've seen:

1. *Many people, including myself, try a "fat-free" diet using "fat-free" foods, which often defeat the purpose of healthy eating.*

Since a food is labeled "fat-free," this often signals that you can eat lots of this product, from cookies to snack foods, and still not get fat. Not true.

Too much of any food—even good foods—can still put on pounds because the excess is converted to fat in the liver.

2. Secondly, I'm not convinced that "fat-free" foods really work.

Our bodies seem to metabolize the fat-free foods as though they are the original high-fat food. Remember, food producers are not often nutritionists; they don't make any guarantees when they write "fat-free" on a label. There is no research or double-blind studies that prove any of these products work.

3. Food processors have eliminated the fats from these foods, and replaced them with sugar. White sugar is stored as fat.

When it comes to weight loss, you have to look at the big picture. Don't just choose foods for what they don't have—fat. Often fat-free foods are high in sugar, chemicals, preservatives, and even damaged fats. Limiting the amount of fat is important, but eating vegetables, fruits and whole grains is equally important. Eat foods for what they do have: minerals, vitamins, fiber and nutrients to help fat burning.

4. Fat-free eating is not as healthy as low-fat eating.

Many people, in their sincere desire to reduce fat in their diet, cut out fat completely, which is dangerous! I've discovered that a no-fat diet causes people to have dry hair, skin, and nails. When they start consuming some of the right fats, these conditions leave. People get healthier and lose weight by eating some fat—vegetable oils, nuts, seeds, and animal foods.

Do Fats Make Us Fat?

Some do and some don't. It all depends on the type of fat. The right fats can help you burn fat! Fats assist the liver to metabolize fats properly. In his book, Udo Erasmus says that a woman lost weight just by adding flaxseed oil to her daily diet:

> W3 fatty acids, which increase metabolic rate, can be used for weight loss. One woman in California lost 80 pounds of excess fat by adding 3 tablespoons per day of fresh flax oil to her dietary program. She had been eating relatively nutritious foods for some time, without

effect. The addition of flax oil was the missing key for her. Weight watchers may find it hard to believe, but here is a fat (actually an oil) that can make fats burn more rapidly. The story illustrates the importance of knowing the difference between killing and healing fat. The right kind of fat can help you lose weight.[1]

Fats help you *lose* fat. Eating a small amount of fat at every meal helps slow down the absorption of carbohydrates.

We Need the Good Stuff

Everyone is familiar with the term essential amino acid. This means there are certain amino acids that our body doesn't make, that we must obtain from outside sources—our diet. The same is true of fats. Some fats are essential because they are not made by the body, but are required by food or supplementation. We desperately need some good fat!

When your body is fat-starved, you get hungry, overeat, and binge on carbohydrates and sweets. Many people think they have a "sweet tooth," when in fact, they may have a "fat tooth." Often when they think they want sweets what they really want is fat. For example, people crave chewy cookies, flavored yogurt, and double-chocolate ice cream. The first ingredient in the label may be sugar, but the second ingredient is fat.

According to author, scientist Brian Scott Peskin, virtually all of us are deficient in the good types of fats because the typical American diet doesn't include them. What we are experiencing in America is a major essential fatty acid (EFA) deficiency! He reports that:

> - It is estimated that 95% of Americans are deficient in EFAs.
>
> - EFAs are removed from processed foods.
>
> - Six months of consistent EFA supplements are usually required before the body develops an adequate reserve.[2]

Where Do We Get Good Fats?

Omega 3 fatty acids are found in all fish, especially cold-water fish, such as salmon, mackerel, sardines, cod, and tuna. The best plant source of Omega 3 is flaxseeds and flaxseed oil. They need to be refrigerated because they are sensitive to light and can become rancid easily.

Omega 6 fatty acids are found in sesame, safflower, corn, and olive oils. While it's good to include Omega 6, a balance of the Omega 3/6 is also important. It's easier for most people to get Omega 6 oils, found in olive oil, so the Omega 3's are more important as a supplement. One to two tablespoons daily of flaxseed oil is a good daily recommendation.

Most of our cell membranes are made of fat. Fat is required for good cellular structure and nutrient absorption. I've recommended good fats for clients who have had arthritis, asthma, PMS, allergies, and skin problems. These good fats also:

- Boost the immune system
- Carry and store fat-soluble vitamins A, D, E, K (for skin and blood clotting)
- Are necessary to make healthy hair, skin, and nails
- Are vital for a healthy immune system
- Are required to build hormones to assist in the treatment and prevention of PMS and other hormonal problems
- Are an excellent source of energy
- Help you handle stress better
- Reduce food cravings and help you feel satisfied
- Can lower cholesterol and triglycerides
- Increase good cholesterol
- Decrease bad cholesterol
- Decrease triglycerides
- Reduce the tendency to form blood clots in arteries
- Decrease total cholesterol, both HDL and LDL
- Can help you lose weight

Fats and Disease

Did you know that approximately one hundred years ago, heart attacks were scarce in the United States? In the early 1900s only about 3 percent of us died from heart disease. Today, nearly half of our population has some type of heart disease. Wait a minute. Realize what we were eating in the early 1900s: fresh, whole foods, meat, butter and even lard! So why weren't there more heart attacks?

It's not enough to know the type of oil you are consuming. How it is processed can make it a fat that will either heal or harm your body. Brian Peskin reports that around the 1930s, "Americans switched from eating butter and other natural fats and oils to highly refined unsaturated oils, margarine and hydrogenated shortening."[3] That's when the rate of heart disease increased.

Two Types of Processing

To understand the correlation between diet and heart disease, let's stop for a moment and look at two ways that oils are processed.

There are basically two types of oils: unrefined, or cold-pressed oils, and refined oils. I recommend natural, cold-pressed, unrefined oils because they go through the least amount of processing. These oils are still dark with possibly some sediment. They taste and smell like the original product. They are rich in nutrients, including vitamin E, which helps to protect the oil from rancidity. These are generally called "cold-pressed," which means the oil has been pressed but no solvents have been used. The heat generated in this type of extraction is very mild compared with that of the high-processed oils.

A Great Oil

Olive oil has been a staple for five thousand years. Populations who use olive oil have a much lower incidence of heart disease and strokes. One reason is that olive oil is the richest monounsaturated fat, and it lowers the LDL cholesterol.

There are three types of olive oil: extra-virgin, virgin, and pure. Extra-virgin means the oil was pressed without further refinement. It is just filtered, and is the least refined. I prefer this type, but the flavor is strong. Virgin olive oil is simply filtered and has a milder taste than extra-virgin. Pure olive oil is a blend of refined olive oil and extra virgin or virgin olive oil. All of these unrefined oils are found in most health food stores. However, some "pure" and "light" olive oils found in the supermarket may be processed with the use of solvents so when buying these oils in the supermarket, I recommend getting the least refined ones (extra-virgin).

The Making of Bad Fats

Refined oils, on the other hand, are quite different from the original product. Refinement means that the oil is clear, odorless, and almost completely devoid of nutrients.

First, the oil is washed with sodium hydroxide. Then caustic sodas are added. Next, they filter the oil through bentonite or other clay to bleach it and remove minerals and color components like chlorophyll. Then the oil is heated to deodorize it. Finally, the oil is hydrogenated to stabilize it (preventing separation of the oil and extending the shelf life.)[4]

Unfortunately, all the chlorophyll, lecithin, Vitamin E, copper, magnesium, calcium, and iron have been processed out, and the product has little nutritional value. On top of this, preservatives (BHA and BHT) are added to keep it from going rancid. But it still is 100 percent fat and is now indigestible! These oils aren't so slick after all.

Trans Fats Are Damaged Fats

Trans fats are fats that have been altered or damaged by high heat. These are a man-made type of fat not found naturally. Processors hydrogenate (add hydrogen molecules) vegetable oils under high heat. What would normally be a liquid oil now becomes solid at room temperature. In other words, your liquid vegetable oil is saturated—a good example is margarine. Eating processed oils like this only confuses your body, which thinks it's a saturated fat, yet tries to use it as an essential fat. Brian says: "An adulterated EFA is not an EFA."[5]

What is the result of eating these altered or damaged fats? These trans-fatty acids not only raise the bad LDL cholesterol level, just like saturated fat, but they also lower the good HDL cholesterol. They hinder your body's ability to use the fat-soluble vitamins, they add to the load of our already overworked liver, and they even cause an essential fatty acid deficiency. What's worse, they hinder weight loss.

Earlier we mentioned that trans fats are linked to heart disease. Again, Brian Peskin reports, "Trans-unsaturated fat, as the man-made stuff is called, is *14 times more potent as a disease risk factor* than the saturated fats the public has been warned about for years—the kind in marbled beef, butter, and cheese."[6]

After reading Brian Peskin's book, *Beyond the Zone,* he will challenge you to rethink everything you have learned about what fat is really bad and what is good. "Maybe it is the lack of EFAs — *not* the cholesterol or fats in eggs, cheese, and steak — that causes the problems."[7]

Good Fats Keep Your Blood Thin

Another interesting fact is that "As early as 1929, it was known that omega 6 promoted naturally 'thinner blood,' along with increasing energy levels."[8]

He explains that thin blood means the platelets don't stick together, an important function for preventing heart attacks and strokes. Natural, essential fats keep the molecules from clumping together! If we had more essential oils, we would have healthier blood and decrease our risk of heart disease. Peskin says:

> Artificially lowering cholesterol levels with drugs disrupts the body's automatic control system. That's why we often see a multitude of negative side effects in other areas when taking drugs. That's why you may wish to read the drug's 'package insert,' so you can be aware of the possible side-effects. Why must we be so frequently reminded that we can't fool Mother Nature?[9]

If our heart problems are linked to an increase in trans fats and a deficiency in essential fats, wouldn't a better and safer approach be to dump the trans fats and start taking essential fats? And one final point from Peskin about weight loss and fats:

> Virtually all research is conducted on test subjects who are EFA-deficient! Obesity is a symptom of EFA deficiency—just as the disease scurvy is a symptom of severe vitamin C deficiency.[10]

Where Do You Get Trans Fats?

Trans or damaged fats are found in margarine, shortening, mayonnaise, and baked goods containing hydrogenated oils and are commonly called "hydrogenated" or "partially hydrogenated" fats. These include breads, cookies, cakes, potato chips, corn chips, taco shells, all commercial vegetable oils, commercial peanut butter, and all fried foods.

Unfortunately, most restaurants use either processed heat-treated vegetable oils or hydrogenated vegetable margarine or both. To add insult to injury, they heat them over and over.

Where's the Fat in Fat-Free Foods?

My friend June and I would occasionally sit down and eat a fat-free chocolate cookie, wondering what in the world was in them. An article in the *Nutrition Action Healthletter* gives some answers:

> ...the Center for Science in the Public Interest (CSPI) has petitioned the Food and Drug Administration (FDA) to require that trans fat be included not just in the Total Fat number on food labels (as it is now), but in the Saturated Fat number as well. That way, consumers would be able to see how much artery-clogging potential any fat had.
>
> The FDA limits the amount of saturated fat in foods that make a 'no-cholesterol' or 'low-cholesterol' claim. But it sets no limit on trans fat. If the agency counted trans along with saturated fat, it would be illegal for products like Nabisco Oreos or Wheat Thins to call themselves 'no-cholesterol.'
>
> Our conclusion: Unsuspecting consumers—some under doctors' orders to cut artery-clogging fat to reduce their risk of heart disease—are being broadsided by foods that are far more damaging than they appear to be.[11]

The Great Debate: Margarine or Butter?

Margarine, shortening, and spread blends are all hydrogenated. Studies have shown that margarine actually coats the stomach wall, rendering foods indigestible. Imagine that!

In *Nutrition Made Simple,* Certified Nutritionist Robert Crayhon says:[12]

Margarine, vegetable shortenings, and all hydrogenated oils:
- Raise total cholesterol levels 20-30%
- Lower HDL cholesterol and raise LDL cholesterol.
- Decrease quality of mother's breast milk by lowering its fat content.
- Promote inflammation.
- Create higher levels of circulating insulin and may cause diabetes.
- Increase the number of fat cells and promote obesity.
- Reduce the ability of the body to rid itself of toxins, carcinogens, and drugs.

- Dangerously alter the function of cell membranes throughout the body.
- Decrease immune function.

Butter Is the Winner!

Butter is better than margarine even though it is higher in cholesterol. You can safely use butter in *small* amounts if you don't heat it. But skip the butter if you are watching your cholesterol. Stay away from palm oil, coconut butter, and products like Crisco. A good replacement for margarine can be made by mixing equal amounts of butter with olive oil.

What About Fake Fats?

Fat substitutes like Olestra are becoming popular. But are these products really helping us win the war over weight? The label contains warnings about possible digestion problems (loose stools and abdominal cramping), saying that it may inhibit the absorption of vitamins, and recommends using it in moderation. You may have heard that it can cause "anal leakage." Does this sound normal or healthy? I'm thinking, what's the point? If we could eat everything in moderation, why would we need fat substitutes?

Olestra is literally indigestible. It tastes like fat, and adds no calories—what a dream food, right? Wrong. You already know how important it is that your foods be digested and absorbed. So what is the potential problem with Olestra? It's toxic. Our bodies are so smart! They know a foreign invader imposing as food when they see it. These fats are toxic and instead of promoting health, they go against your body's normal functioning. Why not work *with* the body, the way it was designed to work, rather than work *against* it with fake fats? Besides, a little bit of the right healthy fat can help you reach your fat-loss goals!

Too Little, Too Much and Just Right

In chapter 3 on digestion, I mentioned that if you are deficient in lipase, the fat digesting enzyme, then you will have trouble digesting fats. So before you eat healthy fats, make sure you can *digest* them. Start with a conservative one tablespoon daily, or 10-20 percent fat in your diet. (See the chart in chapter 18.)

What Can I Do?

1. Read labels. Hydrogenated oils are found in most convenience foods. Label reading is tricky. Just because the label says "all vegetable" oil does not mean it's healthy. It depends on what oil they used and whether or not it's been hydrogenated. Avoid foods that contain hydrogenated or partially hydrogenated oils. Foods that are "cholesterol-free," "low-cholesterol," "low-saturated-fat," or "made with vegetable oil" aren't necessarily low in trans fat. "Saturated-fat free" foods are low in trans fat.

   Avoid oils packaged in a clear bottle. Sunlight can penetrate and the oil will go rancid. Buy them in dark brown bottles. Avoid oils that are odorless and tasteless. These are very refined. Natural oils have flavor.

2. Cut back or eliminate foods made from processed oils: chips, crackers, cookies, pastries, and other processed foods. Get rid of all synthetic or plastic fats. Switch from all margarine to butter. Every type of hydrogenated margarine is plastic! Use extra-virgin olive oil, Pam spray with olive oil (pump), flaxseed oil (don't fry) and small amounts of real butter.

3. Make "better" butter by combining equal parts of real butter with cold-pressed olive oil. Mix well together and use as a spread. Use Nasoya salad dressing (made from tofu). Use Spectrum canola mayonnaise or Lite canola mayonnaise.

4. Stop buying foods that contain bad fats, especially commercial mayonnaise and hydrogenated cooking oils. If you want to become serious about weight loss, damaged fats must be substituted with healthy alternatives like cold-pressed oils and small amounts of good old-fashioned butter.

FOODS TO ELIMINATE

Margarine and fake fats
Deep-fried foods
Chicken-fried steak
French fries
Onion rings
Corn dogs
Egg rolls
Fried potato skins
Fried doughnuts
Hush puppies
Cookies, cakes, pies made with shortening or hydrogenated oils
Breads with hydrogenated oils or fats
Candy bars with hydrogenated oils
Mayonnaise
Crackers and snack foods with hydrogenated oils

For more information, I recommend *Get the Fat Out* by Victoria Moran, *Beyond the Zone* by Brian Scott Peskin, *Fats That Heal/Fats That Kill* by Udo Erasmus, and *Your Fat is Not Your Fault* by Carol Simontacchi, C.C.N., M.S. All of these books are listed in the Bibliography.

I am no longer interested in eating fat-storing, artery-clogging, sickness-producing foods. I love wholesome, natural foods that help me burn fat!

Protei
Much Is Enough:

Mary started her dieting journey following a high-protein diet. It worked for awhile, but she later gained all her weight back. She learned about juicing for health and weight loss and tried that for awhile. The weight she lost found her again! After trying so many seemingly opposite approaches to weight loss, it's no wonder Mary was confused, frustrated and wanted to give up! Let's clear up some confusion about protein.

Saturated Fat Is Still Bad

According to the United States Department of Agriculture, beef consumption increased 75% between 1900 and 1980. "The Dietary Goals for the United States," stated: "The over-consumption of fat, generally, and saturated fat in particular, as well as cholesterol...have been related to six of the ten leading causes of death: heart disease, cancer, cerebrovascular disease, diabetes, arteriosclerosis, and cirrhosis of the liver."[1] For some time we have known that saturated fat is linked to many diseases. Most animal protein contains fat. So what is a good protein and how much is too much?

We Need Some Protein Daily

Protein stimulates the release of glucagon, the fat-burning hormone that helps your body burn stored fat. Proteins build muscle, bone, cartilage, and skin. They are needed to make new hair and nails, replace worn cells, and regulate the body's functions and fluids. Having adequate protein also boosts your metabolism. However, many of my clients have given up protein because it's to high in fat. Some of them eat too much protein. Again, balance is the key. In this chapter, I want to discuss where we get it and what happens if we eat excessive amounts of protein. We'll also see how meat processing methods can affect protein. Protein is the 's main source for growth and tissue repair and is made up of compounds called amino acids. There are twenty of these cute little body builders; eleven of them can be manufactured in the body; the remaining nine must be obtained from food. Protein is not stored and must be replenished daily. Unfortunately, most of the popular protein foods are also high in fat. (You know, like those juicy, plump hamburgers.)

Where Do We Get Protein?

All animal foods like dairy, milk, meat, and eggs provide all of the essential amino acids and make a complete protein. Grains, vegetables, and legumes (beans, lentils) contain protein but lack or are low in one or more of the essential amino acids. However, if you combined the beans and grain together, they form a complete protein containing all the amino acids. (See the chart at the end of this chapter that shows you how to put vegetarian proteins together to make complete proteins.)

Soy protein is a great substitute for meat. (I gave some health benefits for soy at the end of chapter 11. You'll learn more about soy foods in chapters 17-20.)

Vegetarian Bodybuilders?

Bill Pearl, three-time Mr. Universe winner, is well known as a vegetarian bodybuilder. In his book, *Getting Stronger,* Bill reports: "Lying on my couch in my living room, I was having a hard time clenching my fists, wondering what medication I could take for the pain in my elbow and knee joints. I also had high-blood pressure, high cholesterol, and high uric acid. I ate lots of meat, cheese, and dairy products for years until a doctor told me to cut back on fats and sugar."

Bill and his wife, Judy, gave up red meat. Later, eating chicken at a chicken take-out restaurant, he found a growth on the chicken meat. When he discovered that the growth was due to the female hormones producers fed the chickens, Bill and Judy gave up chicken too. As he replaced meat with fertile eggs, fresh fruits, and vegetables, fresh nuts and seeds, whole grains, brown rice, baked potatoes, and low-fat dairy products, he noticed a great improvement in his health. He believes it's a myth that you have to eat meat to have big muscles. And that's from a three-time winner of Mr. Universe titles.[2]

Problems With Excess Protein

In chapter 1, I gave some cautions about the high-protein diet for weight loss. Here are some additional concerns.

1. Excess protein can cause gout. Protein contains high levels of uric acid. Your body can only eliminate about 8 grams of uric acid a day, but the average piece of meat contains 14 grams. Uric acid builds up in the bloodstream, sneaks out of the bloodstream, and if it is not removed from the blood, the excess builds up in the joints and tissues. This later creates gout or kidney problems.

2. Excess protein can make you fat! Four ounces of ground chuck contains 23.9 grams of fat, enough fat for a whole day (and we haven't even touched those French Fries yet). Plant proteins are lower in fat and lack saturated fat altogether. Of the 67 calories in an egg, 80 percent are from fat. One serving of lentil and rice contains 292 calories which is 18 percent fat.

3. Excess protein pulls calcium from the bones. This can cause osteoporosis, where teeth become soft and bones become weak. Meat is a high-acid food and in order to maintain the proper pH balance, your body pulls its reserves of an alkaline buffer—the mineral of choice is calcium. So the more meat you eat, the more calcium your body needs. That's why many high-protein diets recommend a calcium supplement. When your body runs out of calcium reserves, it pulls it from your bones.

4. Additionally, the lack of fiber from eating excess protein can cause constipation. Many high-protein diets recommend no carbohydrates or as few as 20-40 grams daily. Complex carbohydrates are our best form of fiber too. There is no fiber in animal foods or dairy, but there are all types of fibers in vegetables, whole grains, and beans.

5. Excess protein is one reason that the average cholesterol level of Americans is 210. The combination of high cholesterol and high saturated fat make animal foods artery-clogging and fat-depositing. Vegetarians who eat no meat or dairy have a cholesterol count as low as 125 and have less risk of heart disease. (See *Eat More, Weigh Less* by Dr. Dean Ornish.)

6. Excess protein can hurt the heart. If cholesterol and a high-fat diet are the key culprits in heart disease, why haven't we seen more of a reduction in our number one disease killer? In spite of all the low-cholesterol, fat-free foods, heart disease still causes 42 percent of all deaths in the United States.

For thirty years, Dr. McCully, author of *The Homocysteine Revolution*, has worked to prove his theory on the real reason for heart disease: food processing which causes a deficiency of B vitamins. In my practice alone, I've seen that the B vitamins is the single most common deficiency among my clients.

Dr. McCully's bottom line is that these deficiencies of the water soluble B vitamins lead to a buildup of homocysteine, an amino acid that triggers heart disease.

He doesn't suggest that Americans just take their B vitamins and *still* eat cholesterol and fat! Switching to a diet rich in fresh fruits and vegetables is vital. If you have a high-protein intake from animal sources, you definitely need *more* B vitamins. A good recommendation is to take a B vitamin complex and 400 mcg. of Folic Acid daily. (I recommend Cataplex B and Folic Acid/B12 by Standard Process.) Do not buy a synthetic B complex since they are not as effective, and can hinder the healing process.

In his book, *The China Project: Inside Our Living Laboratory,* T. Colin Campbell, Ph.D. states: "In China only 10% of protein is meat protein, where here a whopping 70% comes from meat and milk products."[3]

"Only four in every 100,000 males under age 65 in China die of heart disease each year, while 67 out of 100,000 die in the U.S."[4]

Dr. Campbell's *China Project* also names several diseases that can be prevented or either improved by a semi-vegetarian or vegetarian diet: osteoporosis, obesity, high cholesterol, heart disease, breast cancer, lung cancer, and prostate cancer.[5] He also says that the highest rates of breast cancer occur in the countries where people eat the most meat.[6]

7. Another risk of excess protein is simply the low quality of food. Many Americans love to eat pork in the form of sausage, bacon, and hot dogs. Yet we all know the warning about trichinosis and tapeworms. I've seen the blood of people who eat large amounts of pork, and it's loaded with microscopic bacteria.

We haven't even touched on how meats are prepared for the consumer. If you eat meat, cut out pork, veal, luncheon meats, ham, bacon, and sausage. Smoked, processed, and so-called luncheon meats are high in fat, and saturated fat as well. Additionally, they contain dangerous sodium nitrate and nitrites which have been linked to various types of cancer.

I recommend that you stick with the whole chicken or turkey so you know exactly what you are getting. Buy organically grown meat—that is, meat raised without the use of hormones or antibiotics.

Is Fish Healthy?

Fish is a healthy alternative to beef. Some research shows that eating fish boosts the immune system and circulatory system. The Greenland Eskimos eat a diet rich in cold-water salmon, yet they have little heart disease. Salmon is high in Omega 3 fatty acids, which keep blood from clotting and prevent heart attacks. Cold-water fish like salmon, mackerel, haddock, trout, perch, red snapper, and tuna have the highest amounts of Omega 3.

Even our fish waters can be polluted. Problems with DDT, a carcinogen, and PCB's are rampant. When possible, find the safest source of fish. If you eat canned salmon, pour off the liquid, which is a vegetable fat.

Shellfish are higher in cholesterol and have a poor filtration system, which means they can retain toxins and, therefore, are not recommended for regular consumption either.

You Don't Have to be a Vegetarian

Does this mean you have to give up red meat (and grow a beard and live in a commune)? One big difference between healthy meat-eating cultures and ours is the absence of processing (drugs, hormones, etc.) of animal products. Small amounts of *healthy* meats can be extremely beneficial. (For vegetarians, see chapters 17 and 18 for more about soy protein.)

If animals were raised naturally, with fresh air and light, exercise and a healthy grass diet, probably the types of processing methods would not be necessary, and these foods would retain more of their natural fats, proteins, and enzymes.

Got Milk?

I, like you, grew up drinking milk. Our meals were not complete without a tall glass of milk. Once a week, my father took us all out for ice cream—this was years before we realized how much fats make us fat! I loved milk shakes. But when I stopped drinking milk, I became healthier. I was not successful at weight loss until I eliminated milk and cheese completely.

Milk Has Changed

Back when cows grazed on food that came from untreated soil, milk had a neutral or alkalizing effect on us. As time went on, cows ate a diet of higher protein content, which meant greater milk production. However, milk from high protein-fed cows has an acidifying affect on us. Since milk is now an acid-producing food, the body has to use its calcium mineral reserves to neutralize the acid, just as with meat.

Since our milk is homogenized, this makes milk a processed food. Scientist Brian Peskin has a chapter in his book *Beyond the Zone,* entitled, "Milk: Does It Really Do a Body Good?" Brian believes that homogenization of milk is a possible contributing factor to arterial damage. The homogenization process extends the shelf life of milk, but the xanthine oxidase (XO) in milk attacks the arterial wall, leaving it damaged and weakened. This is a possible explanation for how arterial plaque starts. Brian says cutting back to skim milk or non-fat milk doesn't eliminate the problem, because there is still XO in it. Butter, however is not homogenized, but cheese is.[7]

Traditional cultures eat very little dairy products and when they do, it is usually in the form of yogurt, cottage cheese, buttermilk and kefir, all a type of fermented foods, which makes the milk far easier to digest. Most people of Oriental or African descent can't digest dairy products very well.

Why Don't Chinese People Get Osteoporosis?

In *The China Project,* Dr. Campbell reports: "Although most Chinese consume little if any dairy and ingest low amounts of calcium in general, they appear to be not at higher risk of osteoporosis."[8]

All things being equal, if we are the number one milk-drinking nation, then why do we have the highest incidence of osteoporosis? First, the pasteurization process transforms organic calcium into inorganic calcium. Secondly, as with meat, your body needs to pull calcium from your bones to neutralize the acid. Adequate calcium can help prevent osteoporosis.

Do You Want to Grow Fast?

Finally, milk contains powerful growth hormones that are designed to help a calf grow from ninety pounds at birth to about one thousand pounds two years later. At that rate, a typical eight-pound baby would weigh about eighty-nine pounds in two years.

Have you ever wondered why American children physically mature so fast compared with other cultures? Dr. Campbell sheds some light on the subject of protein and development in his book, *The China Project.* He shares evidence that our bodies should reach puberty much later than we do.

> In countries that follow a predominantly vegetarian diet, puberty would occur at a much later age. Chinese girls reach menstruation usually when they are 15 to 19 years old, quite a bit later than the 10 to 14 that is average in the U.S. What is the cause of this rather dramatic difference? It has to do with what girls eat. Diets high in fat, calories, and animal protein hasten the start of menstruation by accelerating growth.
>
> Young girls are rightly proud of their first periods, as a sign of their womanhood. But the price can be high when this step into adulthood comes too early. The earlier the beginning of menstruation the greater the likelihood of developing cervical as well as breast cancer... What can we do to protect our daughters? Provide a diet low in fat and animal products, and high in vegetables and grains![9]

Another Opinion About Milk

Dr. John McDougall calls milk "liquid meat." Most of the nutrients for which milk is drunk are easily obtained from vegetable foods. Here are some hazards associated with dairy products according to McDougall:[10]

1. Dairy products are the leading cause of food allergies.
2. After the age of four years, most people naturally lose the ability to digest the carbohydrate known as lactose found in milk.
3. Dairy products may contain unsafe levels of environmental contaminants.
4. Dairy products can be contaminated with disease-causing bacteria such as salmonella, staphylococci, and E. coli.
5. The amount of calcium present in the diet has little effect on the quantity of calcium that is eventually taken into the body. High-calcium diets have also been implicated by some investigators as a cause of calcium kidney stones.

6. Low-fat products suffer from the same nutritional inadequacies as their whole-fat counterparts: complete lack of dietary fiber and deficiencies of vitamins and minerals.
7. Infants who are fed whole cow's milk or skim milk as a large part of their diet can develop a nervous system susceptible to disease later on in life.

Another interesting book about milk is called *Don't Drink Your Milk!* by Dr. Frank A. Oaski. He gives the medical facts about the world's most overrated nutrient—a very compelling study about milk, its history, and hazards. It's required reading for anyone with allergies.

Skin Problems Clear Up

Several years ago I met a woman named Karen. She told me that she had psoriasis and had been going to a dermatologist (and taking medications) for twenty years. But she read an article that persuaded her to stop drinking dairy products and eating products containing wheat. In four months, nearly 75 percent of her skin problems disappeared! She couldn't believe that after taking all that medication for so long, the problem could be solved so simply. Over the past twenty years, I've met dozens of people with similar testimonies.

What About Cheese?

You probably know that whole milk and two-percent milk are high in saturated fat and cholesterol. Cheese is far more concentrated than milk. It takes four to five quarts of milk to make a pound of cheese. Many of my clients feel that cheese causes them to have constipation. Cheese is simply artery-clogging, saturated fat. Each ounce of full-fat cheese has four to six grams of saturated fat. Most cheese is heat treated and contains damaged fats. Additionally, many people are unknowingly allergic to milk and cheese or lactose intolerant, and find them hard to digest. I've helped many people lose weight, and many times adding even a little dairy can hinder weight loss. If you are really sincere about losing weight, I recommend that you eliminate all dairy products for six weeks. Following that, eat small amounts of "pre-digested" milk products like yogurt and kefir.

What Can I Do?

1. Read labels. Stick with whole meats such as a whole chicken breast or whole turkey breast. That way you know exactly what you are getting.

2. Cut back or eliminate your consumption of red meat, processed luncheon meats, and high-fat dairy.

3. Substitute. Rather than worry so much about getting enough protein, get quality protein. Wild, or organically raised and drug-free animal proteins like fish, game, free-range poultry, organic beef, and lamb are good choices. You can find "organically" grown, free-range meat at your health food store. (Free-range means the animals have not been penned and have not been injected with harmful hormones.) Look for nitrate-free meat products. Some grocery stores carry lean, hormone-free buffalo meat. Consider using soy substitutes that really look and taste like meat. (More in chapters 17 and 20.)

Switch from processed cheeses to natural cheeses, which don't have artificial colorings.

Order your burgers and salads without cheese.

For flavoring only, try Parmesan, Romano, Feta, Farmers, goat cheese, low-fat mozzarella and muenster cheeses.

Try alternatives to dairy like rice milk, almond milk, and soy milk, which contain natural calcium.

FOODS TO ELIMINATE

Bacon

Beef jerky

Hot dogs

Ham

Bologna, salami, corned beef, pastrami

Sausage

Turkey pastrami

Whole milk

Two-percent milk

Full-fat cheeses

PROTEIN COMPLEMENTARITY

Whole Grains/ or Seeds	Plus Bean	Equals Grams of Usable Protein
$^2/_3$ cup brown rice	$^1/_4$ cup beans	15
$2^1/_2$ cups brown rice	$^1/_4$ cup soy beans $^1/_2$ cup soy flour 6 oz. tofu	37
1 cup brown rice	$^1/_3$ cup sesame seeds 3 Tbsp. sesame butter	16
$1^1/_2$ cups wheat berries or $2^1/_2$ cups bulgur or 3 cups whole-wheat flour	$^1/_2$ cup beans	46
1 cup corn meal or 6-7 corn tortillas	$^1/_4$ cup beans	14
$^1/_2$ cup sesame seeds or $^3/_4$ cup sesame meal or $^1/_4$ cup sesame butter	$^1/_3$ cup beans	19 11

Taken from *Recipes for a Small Planet* by Ellen Buchman Ewald. Used with permission.[11]

I crave good protein, not greasy hamburgers. It's easy for me to eat the right kind and amount of healthy proteins for my body.

Chapter Sixteen

Do You Have
the Caffeine Blues?

Americans run on caffeine. Americans drink more than half of the coffee produced in the world. Coffee is served everywhere, every day for almost every event. And the average American drinks three cups a day. Additionally, many diet plans include coffee as the morning beverage.

When my clients proudly inform me that they don't drink coffee, they usually say that they drink tea or some type of caffeinated soda or pop.

Sometimes when I ask women about their coffee drinking and weight loss, they say, "Well, of course, I drink coffee. I mean, doesn't it help speed up my metabolism so that I can lose weight? Besides, without coffee, I wouldn't even have the energy to exercise."

Caffeine is used to overcome fatigue and seems to improve mental functioning. I learned to love coffee after living in West Germany for three years. An avid coffee lover, I wanted to give you the good news first.

The Bad News

Caffeine makes the body overproduce insulin (hunger hormone), which can make you hungry. So instead of helping you lose weight, it can actually hinder the weight loss. Coffee contributes to lowering blood-sugar levels, which also causes cravings for refined sugars and fatigue.

For years I've observed both in private counseling and in my weight-loss classes, that the people who quit drinking coffee lose weight much easier than those who don't.

Are You Addicted?

Most of us think nothing about drinking one or two cups of coffee a day. After all, millions of Americans daily wake up to a cup of coffee. Or they drink a soda daily. But are they addicted? The only way to really know if someone is dependent on caffeine is to try getting through a day without it.

Do you know how much caffeine you intake daily? Take a moment and list the type and number of caffeine drinks you take daily:

_____

_____

_____

_____

_____

Here's a general idea of the amount of milligrams caffeine contained in various drinks:

BEVERAGE	MILLIGRAMS
1 cup drip coffee	110-150
1 cup percolated coffee	65-125
1 cup instant coffee	40-110
1 cup decaf	2-5
1 cup black tea	20-50
1 cup Hot Cocoa	2-10
12 oz. Mountain Dew	55
12 oz. Coke	46
12 oz. Diet Coke	45
12 oz. Pepsi	40

How Much Is Too Much?

For years, my general recommendation was for my clients to try to eliminate caffeine and soda completely, especially since I saw the link between weight gain and caffeine. But I didn't know how much was too much.

Stephen Cherniske's book entitled, *Caffeine Blues: Wake Up to the Hidden Dangers of America's #1 Drug,* gives a definite link between the amount of caffeine you drink and your risk of disease.

His bottom line is that if you drink between one- to three-hundred milligrams a day, you are already in a danger zone! (That could be one or two cups for most people.) If you drink between three- to nine-hundred milligrams a day, you are addicted. And if you drink nine hundred or more milligrams a day, your heart disease risk factors are significantly increased. A quick nervous system test: extend your arms out in front of you, palms down. If there is any noticeable trembling, caffeine has damaged your nervous system.[1]

Caffeine Is a Legal Drug

The caffeine in coffee, chocolate, sodas and tea is a stimulant drug. When we can't get our early morning dose of caffeine, we experience symptoms typical of withdrawal from any drug: headaches, anxiety, and the jitters. Caffeine also alters moods and changes behavior, and it has a direct effect on the brain and nervous system. The Department of Health lists caffeine along with nicotine and heroin as an addictive substance.

If you happen to be taking thermogenic herbs or herbs that contain high amounts of caffeine, pay attention to your body. If you are "moving and shaking" while you are not in aerobics class, then something is wrong! Don't think those jitters are shrinking fat cells! The caffeine is stimulating your adrenal glands, which can become exhausted—tired. Then you get to where you don't ever want to do anything!

What About Sodas?

When I grew up, drinking sodas was a treat. Today, it's become a staple. But the most vulnerable consumers are our precious children.

Millions of teenagers are addicted to caffeine in sodas yearly. In a chapter entitled, "The Hard Truth About Soft Drinks," Cherniske links drinking sodas to malnutrition, depression, fatigue, decreased learning skills, childhood obesity, and osteoporosis![2]

On the following page is a list of known links to caffeine and disease. Realize that our children are as vulnerable to these as adults.

OTHER PROBLEMS WITH CAFFEINE

- *Heart problems:* Drinking caffeine is related to heart palpitations and high blood pressure. It's also linked to high-cholesterol levels. Two cups of coffee or more can elevate triglycerides or fat in the blood.

- *Vitamin and mineral deficiencies:* Coffee also interferes with absorption of minerals, particularly iron, the essential mineral that prevents anemia. It also leaches out B vitamins from the body, particularly thiamine, which is needed for stress control. So it adds stress instead of taking it away!

  More importantly, without protection from the water-soluble B vitamins, caffeine raises your homocysteine level. Remember, high levels of the amino acid homocysteine can lead to heart disease. If you drink coffee, you must take extra B vitamins daily for protection from heart disease! Caffeine can speed up the loss of calcium in the body, thus weakening bones and contributing to osteoporosis.

- *Pregnancy:* Women who are pregnant are warned against drinking coffee during pregnancy since the coffee can adversely affect the fetus' brain, central nervous system, and circulation.

- *Breast and uterine fibroids in women:* Most research indicates that there is a direct link between fibroid cysts and caffeine intake. Women see almost immediate improvement when they decrease or cut caffeine out of their diet.

- *Headaches and migraines:* Some people experience headaches frequently while drinking coffee, and other people experience headaches after trying to withdraw from coffee drinking.

- *Irritability and mood swings:* Coffee and sugar both have been shown to cause moodiness and anxiety.

- *PMS:* Coffee is also linked to PMS symptoms in women. It's possible that blood sugar or liver problems are made worse by an increase in caffeine intake.

- *Kidney stones:* Coffee contains oxalic acid, which is another acid that needs to be neutralized by calcium in the body. The calcium released from the bones into the blood system eventually winds up in the kidneys. This excess calcium eventually begins to form deposits—kidney stones.

What About the "Low-Lead" Variety?

Decaffeinated coffee isn't much better because they still use chemicals that are carcinogenic. Poisonous herbicide and pesticide sprays are used to cultivate coffee, and then petroleum-based solvents are used to decaffeinate it. Coffee has been implicated in pancreatic cancer because of the hydrocarbons used in the roasting process. Other chemicals are used to make it instant. All of these chemicals have to be filtered by the liver, which often adds a greater burden.

However, Swiss water-decaffeinated coffee is a healthier alternative. Recently much has been written about the benefits of green and black teas as antioxidants, but be aware that they still contain caffeine, so drink them moderately.

What Can I Do?

I know what it's like to try to quit drinking coffee! I try not to drink it, but occasionally I find myself drifting back in the habit. For example, if I am on a book deadline or I lose a night's sleep, (like the night we watched a tornado come through Tulsa), I tend to grab a cup of coffee myself. How do I get off coffee again? The easiest way for me to get off coffee is to plan to drink something else. What has worked best for me is drinking freshly prepared juices, like carrot, apple, or orange, or on a cold day I'll brew a coffee substitute. But I've had to make a firm mental decision and be convinced (again!) of the value of not drinking it—or I'd find myself going back to the coffee.

One obvious connection I've made is that my cycle is pain-free and fairly normal when I don't drink coffee and miserable when I do!

Here are some other suggestions.

1. Read labels to see how much caffeine you are ingesting daily. Look for non-caffeinated drinks. Organically-grown, water-decaffeinated coffee is a safer alternative to decaffeinated coffee. Non-organic coffee beans are loaded with chemical pesticides.

2. Cut back on the amount of caffeine you take daily. If you drink several cups of coffee or soda, then decrease it by one or two cups.

3. To quit caffeine, wean slowly over two to three weeks. The more coffee you drink, the slower you should withdrawal from coffee.

How to get off coffee: Begin by mixing half coffee with a coffee substitute like a popular coffee substitute, Teecino. Teecino can be brewed in drip coffeemakers, percolators, expresso, or French Press pots. Then gradually reduce until you are drinking just the coffee substitute. I like to brew Teecino in my French Press. Instead of adding milk and sugar, I use a little Stevia and soy milk.

How to get off colas and soda pop: First, cut back the quantity. If you were drinking three or four sodas a day, cut back to one. Next, try substituting apple juice for the sodas. Eventually, shift from fruit juices to water or herbal teas.

How to get off tea: Wean off tea over a few weeks by first making your tea half as strong as you used to make it. Then mix it with a no-caffeine herbal tea. Finally switch over to a totally no-caffeine herbal tea.

Drink lots of pure water to help flush caffeine out of your body.

4. Take additional nutritional supplements. Since caffeine causes you to lose water-soluble vitamins, these supplements will help: B complex vitamins, Antioxidant vitamins A, C, E and selenium, flaxseed oil (good fats), and chromium GTF. The herb Ginkgo Biloba may help you with mental clarity. Additionally, help your liver detox with a liver support product.

Be sure you are eating enough good proteins, healthy fats, and complex carbohydrates. Remember, if you need a caffeine fix in the morning to think clearly or get more energy, you may have low thyroid and need to take L'tyrosine. Try taking 500 mg. on an empty stomach in the morning, and/or three times a day. (*Only* take with your doctor's permission, and do not take if you are are taking any medication.) See chapter 6 on low thyroid for more information.

5. Substitute. There are many "coffee substitutes" that could replace your desire for a hot morning drink. Some brands are: Pero, Cafix, Teecino, Pioneer, and Postem. Raja's Cup is a delicious coffee-like herbal antioxidant tea, which may satisfy your coffee cravings. Republic of Tea and Celestial Seasonings both make delicious, non-caffeinated herbal teas with a variety of flavors.

If you need something hot to drink, try hot water with lemon or maple syrup and/or some type of herbal beverage. Many women and men who have taken my classes have withdrawn from coffee by simply switching over to these drinks.

Your health food store has healthier alternatives to many caffeine products. They carry natural sodas, natural teas, organic coffee, cookies, and snacks made with a natural caffeine-free cocoa.

BEVERAGES AND FOODS TO ELIMINATE

Black Coffee or Tea (except herbal)

All colas including "white" colas, such as Sprite and
  Mountain Dew

Cappuccino

Hot chocolate

Dr. Pepper

Chocolate milk

Chocolate candy bars

Cookies with chocolate or chips

Chocolate malts

Coffee flavored snack foods

Chocolate cake

Chocolate pudding

Brownies and fudge

Cocoa

---

*I choose to eliminate caffeine from my diet. I can
wean myself off caffeine safely. It's not a hard thing.
I feel great when I drink healthy beverages. Even
water never tasted so good!*

PART EIGHT

Go For It!

Who satisfieth thy mouth with good things:
so that thy youth is renewed like the eagles.

Psalm 103:5

Chapter Seventeen

Ten Life Design Principles for Healthy Weight Loss

Okay, here's the chapter that I've been leading up to—the chapter that gives you the principles for eating the right kinds of foods to stimulate fat-burning ability. Chapter 18 helps you determine daily servings and chapter 19 gives the meal plans. Chapter 20 gives you a food shopping list. I can't promise that you'll have the body of Cindy Crawford or Arnold Schwarzenegger, but I can promise that you'll look and feel much better as you begin your journey towards permanent weight loss and fat loss.

See Your Doctor

You have just read several chapters that have possibly explained why you haven't been able to lose weight. If after reading these sections, you suspect there may be a problem, see your medical doctor. Don't self-diagnose. Before we get to the principles, let's look at the purpose behind the principles.

Purpose of the Life Design Eating Plan

The Life Design Eating Plan will get you on your way to healthy, safe weight loss. Plan to follow it for the entire six weeks to fully cleanse your liver and tone your digestive system. You will cleanse your body, without the necessity of strict water or juice fasting and you will break any unhealthy habits or food addictions. This plan will:

1. Get you accustomed to eating planned, healthy meals.
2. Cleanse the *body* of accumulated fats in the body and especially in the liver.
3. Heal your stomach and improve your digestion.

4. Improve elimination.
5. Increase your fat metabolism.
6. Restore proper acid/alkaline balance.
7. Reduce cholesterol.
8. Lower blood pressure.
9. Improve blood quality.
10. Increase energy.
11. Beat cravings and help reverse insulin resistance.
12. Help break addictions to caffeine and sugar.
13. Help balance your blood sugar.
14. Help break the habit of having dessert after meals.
15. Help you change your lifestyle to a healthier one.

Principle One: Support your digestion.

In this book, I've given you many causes for weight gain, but start with digestion because most weight problems start with digestive problems. Nearly everyone needs some support for their stomach, colon, and liver. By improving digestion and especially helping the liver, fat loss is much easier. Most of my clients have lost weight and felt better by taking digestion enzymes, doing a colon cleanse, and supporting their liver. These are lifestyle changes and they take time, so give them time. (See Part Two.)

Principle Two: Drink pure water.

Drink plenty of pure water, (not tap water) at least eight to ten 8-ounce glasses daily. Your body is 60-70 percent water, and you need it to flush out toxins. Did you know you can become dehydrated by drinking only herbal teas, coffee, juice, or sodas? Your body wants water! I recommend putting lemons, limes or orange slices in your water for even better digestion, if you can handle citrus fruits. You can drink less water if you eat plenty of high-water content fruits and vegetables.

Principle Three: Eat light at night.

Try not to eat after 7:00 P.M. You'll lose more fat if you eat the majority of your calories earlier in the day.

Eat at least three meals every day, the last meal being the lightest. To keep your blood sugar level normal, try to start your day with something for breakfast—even if it's a protein drink, fruit with nuts, or juice and nuts. Don't skip meals! Skipping breakfast almost always ensures you'll end up later eating more food to make up for lost calories. Eating your large meal at night helps your body store fat even faster.

When people start eating healthy foods, they sometimes enjoy whole foods so much, that they overeat. All foods—even good ones—turn to fat when taken in excess. Eating light is vital, especially at night. People who eat small amounts of food have better digestion and lose weight easier than people who overeat even healthy foods. Eat when you are really hungry and then stop when the hunger cravings are gone.

Principle Four: Eat healthy snacks.

Your snacks should be protein-fat combinations. Throughout this book, I've discussed what a saboteur sugar is for health and weight loss. We were born with a natural sweet tooth that can be satisfied by eating fresh or dried fruits.

Eat well most of the time, but try not to eat desserts for the first two months. Occasionally, make "special treats" with healthy ingredients. I used to give my clients a day off where they could eat whatever they wanted, but we found this idea worked against them, since the refined white sugar and processed foods set up another cycle of binges and cravings. A better idea is go to a health food store and find more wholesome "healthy" cookies, cakes, snacks and even ice cream, and eat them moderately!

Better yet, make healthy desserts with natural ingredients from your health food store. If you eat a dessert, plan ahead and budget. Eliminate the starch in that meal.

Principle Five: Eat more fruits and vegetables.

One of the most important principles for weight loss is to build your meals around healthy vegetables. Most of us eat salads for lunch only on occasion. We'll have a side order of cabbage slaw with a burger or a carrot salad at the deli. But salads are wonderful—as long as you don't overwhelm them with a high-fat dressing! In a balanced diet of carbohydrates, protein, and fat, vegetables and fruits are your fat-burning staples!

Some vegetables and many fruits satisfy your desire for sweets. Eating more servings of fruits and vegetables will increase your vitamin, mineral, and enzyme intake, especially those important antioxidant vitamins,

A, C, and E. Eat colorful vegetables. Rather than eating a white potato, have sweet potatoes or yams for a good healthy change. Easily digestible fruits and vegetables help keep your energy up and your appetite down.

Overall, eat fewer complex carbohydrates and when you do eat them, get the highest-quality complex carbohydrates like whole-grain breads or oatmeal. Whole grains include oatmeal, barley, brown rice, millet, rye and spelt. Small amounts of wheat products are okay if there is no allergy to wheat.

Principle Six: Eat the right fat.

Eat essential fatty acids in the form of extra-virgin olive oil, flaxseed oil, salmon, tuna, almonds, or evening primrose oil. These oils are required by our body and we must get them from foods. They are vital for weight loss, healthy digestion, and proper hormone functioning. Avoid products with hydrogenated oils (peanut butter, margarine, Crisco), all fried foods, and processed vegetable oils. Avoid saturated fat in the form of red meat. (See chapter 14.)

Principle Seven: Eat high-quality protein.

It's vital that you balance your meals with protein, fats, and carbohydrates. If you don't get enough protein, you may lose muscle mass and gain weight. Vegetarian protein can be helpful and effective.

Used moderately, beans and legumes are excellent sources of protein and fiber. Black beans, lentils and kidney beans are easy to use in recipes and excellent for diabetics. (See chapter 15 to learn how to combine vegetable proteins.)

Nutrition-conscious Americans are now enjoying soy-based alternatives to cholesterol containing meat and dairy. Soybeans are high in protein, low in calories, carbohydrates and fats, high in vitamins, easy-to-digest, tasty, and contain no cholesterol. Soy foods protect your heart, help decrease LDL cholesterol, and help reduce the risk of breast cancer, osteoporosis and post-menopausal symptoms in women.

Soybean products have come a long way since the early '70s where the only available foods were tofu or soybean burgers. Today there are hundreds of imaginative, tasteful, fast-food health foods made from soy: tofu pizza, meatless ground round, burgers, deli slices, tofu lasagna, tofu cheesecake, and so on. (See chapter 20.)

Protein drinks and meal replacement bars can be great supplements, if they aren't high in carbohydrates and sugars! The best protein drinks are ion-exchange whey protein, or soy protein. (See chapter 6.) Read labels; some of them are high in sugar. Take digestive enzymes with them.

Drinking a protein drink once a day is a healthy lifestyle change; drinking them more than once a day may be counter-productive. Drinking only meal replacements three times a day rarely result in permanent weight loss since we were created to enjoy chewing.

Principle Eight: Drink healthy caffeine-free beverages.

During the next six weeks, I recommend that lemon water is your drink of choice. Avoid coffee, soft drinks, black tea and chocolate, which all contain caffeine. Caffeine depletes the body of B and C vitamins, some minerals, and causes anxiety, PMS and mood swings. (See chapter 16.)

Principle Nine: Stay motivated.

Throughout this book, I have written motivational statements to encourage you. Appendix A gives a summary of these statements. I encourage you to stay motivated while trying to lose weight. It's okay to get help! Get a supportive friend or prayer partner so that you can support each other.

Principle Ten: Get regular exercise.

Exercise is vital for health and fat loss. It will help you reverse insulin resistance because it encourages the release of glucagon. I believe we are more motivated to do things for ourselves when we know the benefits. After following the Life Design Nutrition eating plan, you *will* have more energy. Exercise won't be so hard for you.

However, I help my clients get healthy before starting exercise. If you are malnourished, it may do more harm than good. Get healthy and more energy *first*. Then start a regular exercise program. Start with something simple — like walking or aerobics.

Here are 55 benefits to regular exercise.

Exercise helps you(r):

1. Improve your breathing.
2. Improve your circulation.
3. Improve your muscle tone.
4. Decrease your weight.
5. Relieve stress.
6. Spend less time feeling sick.
7. Sleep better.
8. Feel more confident with higher self-esteem and self-worth.
9. Feel more in control of your body.
10. Be more active and productive.
11. Enjoy life with a better attitude.
12. Have more control of your life.
13. Extend your chances of living longer.
14. Have clearer nasal passages.
15. Your skin look more supple and elastic.
16. Your ability to burn fat to be more efficient and increase your metabolism.
17. Replace fat with lean tissue; you will lower body fat and lose inches.
18. Combat depression.
19. Lower your blood pressure.
20. Improve your coordination and balance.
21. Normalize/lower your blood sugar.
22. Increase oxygen to the brain, which makes you more alert and clear thinking.
23. Decrease your appetite.
24. Increase overall flexibility.
25. Improve your ability to fight disease because your immune system is strengthened.
26. Your set point be lowered.

27. Reduce the risks of heart disease.

28. Increase the chance of surviving a heart attack and stroke.

29. Reduce fatigue and increase strength.

30. Improve your posture.

31. Reduce chances of developing varicose veins.

32. Relieve and/or prevent constipation.

33. Decrease your desire for nicotine and other substances.

34. Burn calories more consistently.

35. Strengthen your bones/helps prevent osteoporosis.

36. Remove lactic acid and other poisons from the body.

37. Slow down the aging process.

38. Enjoy a better sex life.

39. Increase your chances of being self-motivated.

40. Improve your relationships.

41. Prevent senility.

42. Achieve lifetime weight control.

43. Increase your HDL cholesterol.

44. Decrease your cancer risk.

45. Improve diabetes management.

46. Lower your resting heart rate.

47. Improve your work performance.

48. Reduce lower back pain.

49. Improve stress management.

50. Reduce anxiety.

51. Increase endurance.

52. Improve your vision.

53. Cleanse the body of toxins.

54. Absolutely improve the overall quality of your life.

55. Have an avenue for a healthy means of escape.

Nutritional Summary

TEN LIFE DESIGN PRINCIPLES

Principle One: Support your digestion.

Principle Two: Drink pure water.

Principle Three: Eat light at night.

Principle Four: Eat healthy snacks.

Principle Five: Eat more fruits and vegetables.

Principle Six: Eat the right fat.

Principle Seven: Eat high-quality protein.

Principle Eight: Drink healthy caffeine-free beverages.

Principle Nine: Stay motivated.

Principle Ten: Get regular exercise.

It's easy to change my diet! I will achieve my weight-loss goals if I don't give up. I love exercise. It's easy to lose weight when I do it right!

Chapter Eighteen

Are You Fit for Life or in the Zone?

Every culture has roots and traditions, many of which revolve around natural, local foods. For Americans, it's different. Ask someone what the Basic Four is and they might reply, "Milk, meat, brownies, and ice cream!" If we look at Americans, we might guess that Sara Lee shaped many of us!

What About Proteins, Fats and Carbs?

For years people have debated about the optimum amounts of these nutrients. I've counseled clients who ate too much protein, especially bacon and sausage. They couldn't lose weight. Their overworked liver couldn't handle that much fat and protein.

I've also counseled vegetarian clients who ate too many carbohydrates. They couldn't lose weight either because excess carbohydrates are stored as fat. How can you determine the right types and amounts of foods to eat?

What's Your Type?

No one person has all the answers to the complex issue of weight loss and nutrition, although many people have many pieces to a complex puzzle. I am extremely grateful for the committed nutritionists and authors whom I have quoted in this book after studying nutrition and weight loss for nearly twenty years. This field is exciting and there is so much more to learn!

Let me begin this chapter by presenting a some additional ideas for diet planning, regarding your blood type and ancestry.

A popular book by Dr. Peter D'Adamo entitled, *Eat Right for Your Type* recommends that people eat according to their blood type. It would be beyond the scope of this book to list his specific diet and supplement recommendations for each blood type. But a general statement would be that he recommends that people with type O blood eat animal protein; people with type A blood make better vegetarians; people with blood type B can do well with dairy, and small amounts of meat and fish; and people with blood type AB seem to do well with yogurt, dairy and eggs.

Some of my clients felt better on his plan, and some didn't. Each plan does eliminate "junk foods," which is healthier for everyone. You may want to consider your blood type a factor in planning your diet.[1] (See the Bibliography section for further information on Dr. D'Adamo's book.)

Where Are You From?

Nutritionist Dr. Patrick Quillin recommends that you consider your ancestry and climate. He says that humans, like all other animals on earth, must pay homage to our origins; we must eat our "factory specification" diet. Trying to run a diesel truck on gasoline would ruin the engine. Many people are trying to run their body on the wrong fuel.[2]

Quillin says that Northern Europeans (Norway, Sweden, Scotland, Ireland, and Denmark) existed on fish and lean wild game during the winter. The cold climate made fruits and vegetables scarce until summer and fall. Most light-haired, light-skinned Northern Europeans ate a diet that included dairy and milk. These people have the enzymes necessary for digesting dairy foods.[3]

People from warmer climates, like central Africa and India, rely on a year-round diet of fresh plant foods.[4] Since these people rarely ate dairy, they often are lactose-intolerant, lacking the enzymes to digest dairy foods. If you are from an Asian, Chinese, or African American background, you probably don't digest milk and dairy products well.

The Life Design Eating Plan:
Bible-Based Whole Foods and Nutrition

My focus is to help you to eat more fruits and vegetables, less processed carbohydrates, get enough protein and fat, and support your digestion.

What would this look like? Think about traditional diets, which are what I called "Bible based," like the Mediterranean Diet or Oriental diets. They include fresh salads with "green" Romaine, spinach or red/green leaf lettuce, sprouts, fresh tomatoes, cucumbers, onions, with an olive oil/vinegar dressing and even some Feta cheese for flavoring. Fish or salmon are often served; nuts, seeds, beans, avocado, tofu or tempeh, and

179

fresh fruits and vegetables are common. An Oriental stir-fry with fresh vegetables and fish or chicken makes a wonderful meal.

What I'm recommending is that we go back to healthy, balanced eating, supplemented with good oils in the form of nuts, seeds, avocados and olive or flaxseed oil. The great thing about eating this way is that you don't have to have lots of recipe books, and you can make creative, healthy salads, vegetables and grilled meats or fish.

Some Carbohydrates Make You Fatter

Let's compare two different meals. Meal One has almost half the carbohydrates as Meal Two, yet both are vegetarian based:

MEAL ONE	CARBOHYDRATE GRAMS
Boca burger	13
Soy Crunch bread	11
Vegetables/salad	6
Total	30 grams
MEAL TWO	**CARBOHYDRATE GRAMS**
Regular vegetable burger	36
Whole-wheat bread	24
Vegetable salad	6
Total	66 grams

Simply by substituting lower glycemic-index carbohydrates (such as soy foods), you can keep the protein, but lower the carbohydrates in a meal. This is tremendously important for people who struggle with carbohydrate sensitivity.

Most vegetable burgers are made from grain and bean combinations, which are higher on the Glycemic Index. For a list of soy protein foods, see "Protein and Fat Content of Vegetarian Foods" at the end of this chapter. If you don't eat eggs, eat tofu, seeds, nuts and legumes. Whole grains are better than pasta.

How Much Do I Need?

In the past, I've used formulas and charts for determining daily servings of foods for my clients. An easier way is to plan meals using the USDA's Food Guide Pyramid, which is a visual representation of how to eat foods relative to each other.

The Food Pyramid is a step in the right direction, but it emphasizes a high-carbohydrate intake, which is too much for most people. It also doesn't show important distinctions like the type of fat, quality of meat, or the difference between white and wheat bread, distinctions which I have made in this book and will explain relative to the Food Pyramid. Under each group, we will make these distinctions, looking at both quality and quantity. Having worked with so many clients who were allergic to dairy products, and sensitive to carbohydrates, I've modified the serving suggestions slightly. The serving sizes are listed at the end of the chapter.

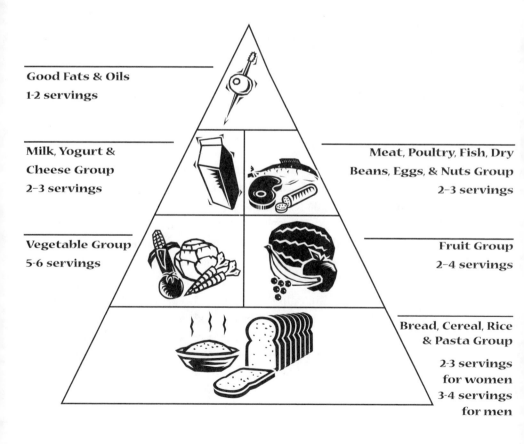

Good Fats & Oils
1-2 servings

Milk, Yogurt &
Cheese Group
2-3 servings

Meat, Poultry, Fish, Dry
Beans, Eggs, & Nuts Group
2-3 servings

Vegetable Group
5-6 servings

Fruit Group
2-4 servings

Bread, Cereal, Rice
& Pasta Group
2-3 servings
for women
3-4 servings
for men

Bread, Cereals, Rice and Pasta Group

1. *Quality:* Choose whole-grain breads and cereals. Refined white breads and pasta can raise your insulin, cause cravings, and weight gain. Also, some carbohydrates are too high in fat for your weight-loss planning. For example, a croissant is about 80 percent fat; a bowl of brown rice is about .5 percent fat.

Wheat can be a problem for many people and may cause gas, bloating and weight gain. (See chapter 7 on allergies.) Try brown rice, or even some unusual grains such as millet or quinoa for a change.

2. *Quantity:* During my early macrobiotic bean-eating, rice-chewing days, I definitely ate six or more servings of carbohydrates a day. I ate whole wheat toast or cereal for breakfast, whole-wheat sandwiches for lunch, and brown rice and vegetables for dinner.

After awhile, my cravings for sugar and carbohydrates became worse. I was eating more carbohydrates and enjoying them less!

Most of my clients report that they can't eat six or more servings of carbohydrates either. When they do, they feel sluggish and tired. Rather than eating 6-11 servings, I recommend eating 2-3 servings for women and 3-4 servings for men. (See the Fiber chart in chapter 13 for help in getting more fiber.) If you are sleepy after eating carbohydrates, then you are eating too many.

Vegetable Group

1. *Quality:* The most important vegetables, such as green leafy vegetables are often overlooked. Canned vegetables lack enzymes. Frozen are better, and fresh is best. The best vegetables are organically grown.

2. *Quantity:* Have you ever heard a wife say to her husband, "Honey, you eat too many salads!" Or, to her children, "Kids, you really have to watch your intake of vegetables." No, if anything, it's the other way around. Husbands, kids, and even many moms don't get enough vegetables! A quick look in shopping carts at any supermarket shows an overwhelming absence of these wonderful foods.

To get 5-6 servings daily, you can eat two large salads consisting of a cup of leafy greens, $1/2$ cup of vegetables, and two or more servings of other vegetables.

Fruit Group:

1. *Quality:* Eat a variety of fresh, low-sugar fruits like apples, pears, peaches, and berries. Canned fruits are lower in enzymes and nutrients; frozen are better, and fresh fruits are best.

2. *Quantity:* I recommend that people eat two fruits a day, preferably fresh fruits. In the summer and spring, fruits make a nice meal along with a handful of raw nuts for protein. Many of my clients have eaten too many fruits, which caused their mineral balance to be off.

Milk, Yogurt and Cheese

1. *Quality:* I've already discussed how processing affects milk in chapter 15. If you drink milk, switch from processed whole milk and 2 percent to skim milk. Better yet, get "organically grown" milk. And skip the cheese. I've never been able to help someone lose weight who ate a lot of cheese! Many of the "lite" varieties of cheese are still 60 percent fat.

2. *Quantity:* Most people easily get two servings of dairy foods every day. They may have milk on their cereal, or yogurt at lunch. If you eliminate dairy, eat more plant foods containing calcium (see the chart at the end of the chapter), and/or take a calcium supplement.

Strict vegetarians (vegans) can replace eggs, milk, cottage cheese, and cheese with tofu, soy milk, and soy cheese.

Meat, Poultry, Fish, Dry Beans, Eggs, & Nuts Group

1. *Quality:* Fish, turkey, beans, and skinless chicken are low in fat. The "Protein and Fat Content of Animal Foods" at the end of this chapter shows you that red meat and hamburgers are too high in fat for regular consumption. Eat poultry, fish or vegetarian proteins including soybeans and other beans. Again, organic meat is preferable in every case.

2. *Quantity:* In counseling people, I've noticed that most men eat too much protein, and many women don't eat enough protein. Men require about 55 grams, and women require about 45 grams per day, which means 2 or 3 servings a day, depending on your size. A common formula for determining your daily number of grams of protein is to divide your weight by 2.2 which gives your weight in kilograms; then multiple that by .8. Remember to try to have some protein at every meal. (Three ounces of meat, chicken or fish equals about 20 grams. See the serving sizes at the end of this chapter.) Athletes and bodybuilders should add 20-30 more

grams of protein a day. The more active you are, the more protein you need. Also, bigger people need more protein.

Good Fats and Oils

1. *Quality:* In chapter 14, we mentioned the difference between good fats (Omega 3) and bad fats (trans fats). The right kind and amount of fat can help you burn fat. Choose non-hydrogenated mayonnaise and salad dressing and skip the fried foods!

2. *Quantity:* People have been more confused about fats than anything else. The low-fat diet has failed, and is even dangerous. We need good fat every day to burn fat and stay healthy. The Mediterranean people eat about 40 percent fat and have little if any heart disease. Add good fat back to your diet, especially if you have been eating a low-fat diet. Eat the good fat, but count the fat grams. The chart in this chapter entitled "Fat Gram Intake Per Weight" shows fat gram totals at 10, 20, and 30 percent of your calories. For weight loss and health, 20 to 30 percent is the safest. Don't be afraid to consume enough good oils, which helps fat-burning.

How Much Should I Eat?

How do you know how many servings to eat? Start with the minimum, eating three meals and two snacks a day. If you find that you are still hungry, then eat more low-fat foods, especially vegetables.

I've included several charts in this book to help you with menu planning. For help computing fats and fat grams, see Appendix F, "Fat Formulas and Fats," and Appendix E, "How To Read a Food Label." For help computing grams of carbohydrates, see "Carbohydrate Grams in Various Foods," at the end of this chapter.

What Are the Serving Sizes?

Bread, Cereals, Rice and Pasta Group:

Serving size: 1 slice bread, 1/2 cup cooked cereal, rice or pasta, 1 cup dry cereal, 1/2 bagel or English Muffin, 3-4 crackers, 1 tortilla, 1 chapati

Vegetables:

Serving size: 1 cup raw, leafy vegetables, 1/2 cup chopped or cooked vegetables, 3/4 cup of vegetable juice

Fruits:

Serving size: 1 piece of fruit, 4 ounces of juice, 1/2 cup canned fruit, 1/4 cup dried fruit, 1 cup berries

Milk, Yogurt and Cheese:
Serving size: 1 cup milk or yogurt, ¹/₂ ounces of natural cheese, 2 ounces of processed cheese, ¹/₂ cup lowfat cottage cheese

Meat, Poultry, Fish, Dry Beans, Eggs, & Nuts Group:
Serving size: 3 oz. poultry, fish or lean meat, 1 egg, ¹/₂ cup beans, 1 oz. nuts

How About Servings for Vegetarians?

Serving size to replace milk, dairy, and meat: 1 cup soy milk, ¹/₂ cup tofu or tempeh, 1 soy burger, 2 soy hot dogs, 3¹/₂ tablespoons of soy protein powder, ¹/₂ cup cooked beans or peas, two tablespoons of peanut butter, ¹/₄ cup (1 oz.) nuts, ¹/₄ cup seeds

FAT GRAM INTAKE PER WEIGHT

Percentage of Fat grams per day at:
10%, 20%, 30%

Weight	Calories	10%	20%	30%	Saturated Fat Grams
100	1100	12	24	36	5-6
110	1210	13	27	40	6-7
120	1230	14	29	41	6-7
130	1430	16	31	47	7-8
140	1540	17	34	51	7-8
150	1650	18	36	55	7-8
160	1760	19	39	58	8-9
170	1870	20	41	62	9-10
180	1980	22	44	66	9-11
190	2090	23	46	69	10-11
200	2200	24	49	73	11-12
210	2310	25	51	77	11-12
220	2420	26	53	80	12-13

PROTEIN AND FAT CONTENT OF VEGETARIAN FOODS

Names of Foods	Grams of Protein	Grams of Fat
Soy Milks:		
Original Extra Edensoy	10	4
Eden Soy Vanilla	6	4
West Soy 100% Original, unsweetened	7	4
West Soy Plus, Vanilla	6	4
West Soy nonfat Vanilla	3	0
Health Valley Soy Moo (fat free)	6	0
Pacific Lite Plain	4	2.5
VitaSoy Enriched Vanilla	6	3
Solair Vanilla Bean	3	2
Other Soy Foods:		
Boca Burger	12	0
Lightlife Meatless Lightburgers	16	1
Lightlife Smart Deli (Roast Turkey Style)	9	0
Lightlife Smart Ground	12	0
Lightlife Smart Dogs	9	0
TofuRella Tofu Cheese	6	5
Yves Veggie Tofu Wieners	9	0
16 oz. Nasoya tofu (firm)	9	5
16 oz. Nasoya tofu (soft)	7	3
Beans, 1 cup:		
Navy beans	14	0
Kidney beans	13	0
Black beans	12	0
Seeds and Nuts, 1 ounce:		
Sunflower seeds	8	15
Almonds	5	15
Walnuts	5	16

PROTEIN AND FAT CONTENT OF ANIMAL FOODS

Names of Foods	Grams of Protein	Grams of Fat
Beef, 4 ounces:		
Ground beef, lean	28	20
Most commercial hamburgers	33	36
Most commercial cheeseburgers	33	45
Fried Fish	22	20
Roast beef	19	20
Poultry, 4 ounces:		
Chicken breast (not fried)	31	5
Chicken breast (fried)	31	12
Turkey meat (not fried)	34	8
Turkey meat (fried)	33	13
Fish, 4 ounces:		
Tuna Fish (packed in water)	15	2
Tuna Fish, (packed in oil)	20	9
Halibut	30	3
Trout	30	5
Haddock	24	1
Dairy, 4 ounces:		
Low-fat yogurt	6	2
Non-fat yogurt	6	0
Milk, whole	8	8
Milk, 2%	8	5
Milk, 1%	8	3
Cottage cheese, low-fat, 1%	14	1

CARBOHYDRATE GRAMS IN VARIOUS FOODS

Food	Amount	Grams of Carbohydrates
Angel hair pasta	2 oz	40
Whole-wheat spaghetti	2 oz.	40
Elbow macaroni	2 oz	34
Whole-wheat lasagna	2 oz.	30
Quick brown rice	1/3 cup	32
Vegetable rice	1/2 cup	32
Wild rice	1/3 cup	15-20
Millet	1/3 cup	34
Cream of Wheat	1 cup	29
Corn meal	1 cup	26
Brown rice	1/2 cup	25
Oat bran	1/3 cup	23
Whole-wheat bread	1 slice	13
Garbanzo beans	1/3 cup	18
Black beans	1/3 cup	16
Split peas	1/3 cup	14
Lentils	1/3 cup	13

*Taken from nutrition labels of Arrowhead Mills products.

CALCIUM CONTENT OF FOODS	
Food	**Calcium (milligrams)**
Milk, 1 cup:	
Skim	315
Low-fat (1%)	315
Low-fat (2%)	315
Whole	290
Yogurt, 8 ounces:	
Plain, low-fat	415
Flavored, low-fat	390
Fruit, low-fat	345
Fruit, whole milk	335
Cheese, 1 ounce:	
Mozzarella, part-skim	205
Natural swiss	270
Natural Cheddar	200
Low-fat cottage cheese, $\frac{1}{2}$ cup	25
Low-fat ricotta, $\frac{1}{2}$ cup	335
Beans:	
Soy milk, 1 cup	200
Tofu, firm, $\frac{1}{2}$ cup	258
Tofu, soft, $\frac{1}{4}$ cup	130
Soybeans, cooked, 1 cup	175
Lentils, cooked, 1 cup	50
White beans, 1 cup	161
Navy beans, 1 cup	128
Vegetables, cooked, 1 cup:	
Broccoli	130
Mustard Greens	100
Spinach	106
Kale	94
Butternut squash	84
Romaine lettuce, 1 cup	20

CALCIUM CONTENT OF FOODS (cont'd.)

Food	Calcium (milligrams)
Fruits and Nuts:	
Calcium-fortified Orange Juice 1 cup	300
Figs, dried (5)	135
Apricots, dried, 1 cup	60
Navel orange, 1 medium	56
Almonds, 1 ounce	75
Sesame Seeds, 1 Tbsp.	100
Fish:	
Sardines $1/_4$ lb.	300
Ocean perch, 4 ounces	156
Blackstrap molasses, 1 Tbsp.	150

I love designing my life so I can eat well and lose weight safely. I take responsibility for what I eat. I love how great I feel when I eat healthy foods.

Chapter Nineteen

The Life Design Six-Week Eating Plan

The following eating plan has helped me stay healthy, lose weight, and keep it off. I don't eat as much food as I used to eat, and I have far more energy. I follow Phase One most of the year. If I put on any weight, I follow Phase Two. The greatest thing about this plan is that you can design it as a lifestyle, as I have safely for many years.

Phase One: The First Three Weeks

This simple plan incorporates animal protein using eggs, chicken, turkey or fish, and/or vegetable protein (soy, beans and rice) depending on your preference (no red meat or pork). Following the guidelines in the previous chapter, eat three meals and two snacks daily. Eat at least two to three protein servings, several vegetable servings (two green salads a day would be great), only two or three servings of carbohydrates, one to two tablespoons of fat, preferably good olive oil, and some fruits. Don't be afraid to eat enough food, especially proteins and fats. Use cottage cheese, non-fat yogurt or kefir for your calcium. If you are really hungry all the time, or you crave sweets and carbohydrates, then try eliminating *all* bread, pasta, rice and refined carbohydrates for the first one or two weeks. You'll be eating fruit, lean protein, and lots of vegetables. During this time, your body will start some gentle housecleaning.

Phase Two: The Three Week Liver Cleanse

Now we want to help cleanse the liver by eliminating saturated fats, so we eliminate all dairy, eggs, and red meat. Many people substitute soy or rice milk for cow's milk. A calcium supplement (1200 mg.) is recommended during these three weeks. Small amounts of fish or chicken are allowed. Lots of fresh, raw fruits and vegetables are recommended, because they are so vital for cleansing the liver. Build your meals with a fresh, green salad, piece of chicken breast and piece of whole-grain bread to keep your blood sugar balanced. (If you are really fatigued, wait until you are well to do the liver cleanse.)

Maintenance and Beyond

Following these six weeks, you can go back to Phase One and safely follow it for the rest of your life. Go to Phase Two if you find yourself falling back into old habits following a vacation or holiday. Remember to limit the amount of fats, even good fats.

Some of my clients feel so good after Phase Two that they now attempt to follow a three-day juice fast. (See your health professional before you start a fast.) Therapeutic fasting with juices is wonderful, and I always recommend that people follow my six-week plan before attempting them. Remember to dilute high-glycemic fruit and vegetable juices, and add barley green or green vegetables. If you juice fast when you are too toxic, you can expect headaches and fatigue. An easier way to fast is with melons and watermelons. Don't juice if you have diabetes or low-blood sugar, either. I don't recommend water fasting at all. A great book on juice fasting is *Juicing for Life* by Cheri Calbom.

About the Recipes

Drawing from the cooking classes that I've taught over the years, I came up with some easy recipes to get you started. The recipes that are starred (*) are listed in the recipe section of this book. (Eating out during either of these Phases can be challenging. See Appendix G for help.)

Phase One: The First Three Weeks

If you don't have hypoglycemia, diabetes, and you are not sugar sensitive, consider eating fruit as a meal with 10 raw nuts or ½ cup yogurt (for breakfast, lunch or dinner). If your energy level doesn't fall from low-blood sugar following a fruit meal, then you probably can handle some fruit. This is especially good in the summer months or a warm climate because fruits are cleansing, easy to digest and satisfy your sweet tooth. Lunch and dinner should include a vegetable, starch and a small amount of protein.

Drink lots of water. Buy several liter-size water bottles and keep in the house, car, or at work. Adding some lemon and a small amount of Stevia makes it tastier. Here is a sample day that includes three meals and two snacks. Lunch and dinner are interchangeable.

PHASE ONE: SAMPLE MEAL PLANNER

Upon arising, have some water or the *Lemon Drink. Have herbal tea or water with meals.

Breakfast

Choose from:

1. *Oatmeal or Oat Bran (with small amount of protein like egg or cottage cheese) OR
2. *Protein Drink or *Protein Drink Smoothie OR
3. Eggs with one slice of whole grain toast and butter OR
4. Fruit and nuts meal (see note on previous page)

Lunch

Try to have a large vegetable dish, animal or vegetable protein and one-half to one serving of a complex carbohydrate.

Choose from:

1. Vegetable salad, grilled chicken strips (or vegetarian protein) and one slice of whole grain bread
2. Stir-fried vegetables, baked salmon (or tempeh or tofu), and one-half of a baked potato
3. Steamed vegetables, turkey breast (or tempeh or tofu), and one slice of bread or a baked yam

Dressing: Make an olive oil, lemon dressing. See the recipe section for healthy salad dressings.

Dinner

Same as lunch. Try to have a large vegetable dish, animal or vegetable protein and one-half to one serving of a complex carbohydrate.

Vegetarian Alternatives: (See chapter 20 and the recipe section for further explanation.)

Choose from:

1. Make the protein drink with soy milk or tofu
2. Make the Tofu "Eggless" Salad
3. Cut tofu in cubes and saute in a stir-fry with vegetables
4. Substitute Boca Burger or Lightlife Meatless Burger for Turkey Burgers
5. Use black beans or chili in place of animal protein
6. Use Fakin' Bacon or grilled tempeh in place of grilled chicken
7. Grate tempeh with a cheese grater, and lightly saute in a small amount of olive oil and use in place of hamburger meat

Snacks

Choose from:

1. Protein Drink or a protein bar
2. One-fourth cup cottage cheese or yogurt
3. Ten raw nuts or handful of seeds

4. Two Wasa bread crackers with 1 slice natural cheese
5. Two Kavli Crispbread with chicken strips and Dijon mustard

PHASE ONE: SEVEN DAYS OF MEALS

Day One
Upon arising, have some water or the *Lemon Drink.
Breakfast
   *Protein Drink or *Protein Drink Smoothie (or fruit if appropriate) OR
   *Oatmeal and one egg or cottage cheese
   Herbal tea or water
Snack: (See page 192 for healthy snack choices)
Lunch
   *Grilled Caesar Chicken Salad OR Caesar Salad with Fakin' Bacon strips
   One slice Whole-grain bread
   Herbal tea or water
Snack: (See page 192 for healthy snack choices)
Dinner
   *Dijon Perch OR *Baked Kidney Beans
   *Greek Salad
   Two rye crackers

Day Two
Upon arising, have some water or the *Lemon Drink.
Breakfast
   *Protein Drink or *Protein Drink Smoothie (or fruit if appropriate) OR
   *Oatmeal and one egg or cottage cheese
   Herbal tea or water
Snack: (See page 192 for healthy snack choices)
Lunch
   Turkey Chili (Shelton's brand from health food store) OR
   *Simple Bean Chili
   *Mexican Taco (Tempeh) Salad
   One slice Whole-grain bread and butter
   Herbal tea or water
Snack: (See page 192 for healthy snack choices)
Dinner
   *Lemon Baked Halibut OR
   *Greek Lentils
   *Classic Mixed Green Salad
   Herbal tea or water

Day Three

Upon arising, have some water or the *Lemon Drink.

Breakfast

*Protein Drink or *Protein Drink Smoothie (or fruit if appropriate) OR
*Oatmeal and one egg or cottage cheese
Herbal tea or water

(Snack: See page 192 for healthy snack choices)

Lunch

Large Vegetable Salad
*Basic Italian Dressing or *Tofu Dijon Dressing
Baked chicken breast or Lightlife Meatless Burger
Three small new potatoes
Herbal tea or water

(Snack: See page 192 for healthy snack choices)

Dinner

Steamed vegetables (carrots, broccoli, cauliflower)
Three ounces fish or chicken (baked or grilled, not fried) OR tempeh
One slice Whole-grain bread
Herbal tea or water

Day Four

Upon arising, have some water or the *Lemon Drink.

Breakfast

*Protein Drink or *Protein Drink Smoothie (or fruit if appropriate) OR
*Oatmeal and one egg or cottage cheese
Herbal tea or water

(Snack: See page 192 for healthy snack choices)

Lunch

*Grilled Caesar Chicken Salad OR Caesar Salad with Fakin' Bacon strips
One slice Whole-grain bread
Herbal tea or water

(Snack: See page 192 for healthy snack choices)

Dinner

*Chicken Oriental Stir-fry OR Stir-fry with Tofu
One-half cup *Basic Brown Rice
*Classic Mixed Green Salad
Herbal tea or water

Day Five

Upon arising, have some water or the *Lemon Drink.

Breakfast

*Protein Drink or *Protein Drink Smoothie (or fruit if appropriate) OR
*Oatmeal and one egg or cottage cheese
Herbal tea or water

(Snack: See page 192 for healthy snack choices)

Lunch

*Herbed Chicken OR Boca Burger on a wheat bun
*Healthy Coleslaw
One baked yam
Herbal tea or water

(Snack: See page 192 for healthy snack choices)

Dinner

*Chicken Cacciatore OR Spicy Black Beans
*Greek Salad
*One slice whole-grain bread
Herbal tea or water

Day Six

Upon arising, have some water or the *Lemon Drink.

Breakfast

*Protein Drink or *Protein Drink Smoothie (or fruit if appropriate) OR
*Oatmeal and one egg or cottage cheese
Herbal tea or water

(Snack: See page 192 for healthy snack choices)

Lunch

*Easy Baked or Grilled Fish OR
*Simple Bean Chili
Cucumber Salad
One slice whole-grain bread
Herbal tea or water

(Snack: See page 192 for healthy snack choices)

Dinner

Shelton Turkey Burger (purchase at health food store)on wheat bun OR
*Boca Burger on wheat bun
Salad of your choice
Herbal tea or water

Day Seven

Upon arising, have some water or the *Lemon Drink.

Breakfast

*Protein Drink or *Protein Drink Smoothie (or fruit if appropriate) OR
*Oatmeal and one egg or cottage cheese
Herbal tea or water

(Snack: See page 192 for healthy snack choices)

Lunch

*Vegetable Chop Suey
*Easy Salmon Bake or Grilled Tempeh
One-half cup *Oriental Wild Rice
Herbal tea or water

(Snack: See page 192 for healthy snack choices)

Dinner

*Chicken Italian Style with whole-grain pasta OR
Spaghetti with Soy Ground Round and whole-grain pasta
*Classic Mixed Green Salad
Herbal tea or water

Phase Two: The Three-Week Liver Cleanse

I encourage you to follow Phase One before you progress to Phase Two. Cleansing diets and modified types of fasting are therapies. I only recommend this liver cleanse for one to three weeks at a time, one to two times a year. It's especially effective to cleanse during the warmer months. Don't try to live on a cleansing diet unless you are working with a health professional, especially if you live in a cold climate. Your body needs to build as well as cleanse.

Again, drink lots of water. Buy several liter-size water bottles and keep in the house, car or at work. Adding some lemon and a small amount of Stevia makes it tastier.

These meals are very simple. You don't need recipes, just have a big salad, steam some vegetables and get some protein.

For optimum cleansing, eliminate or drastically reduce the following which can hinder the healing process:

No white sugar, white flour, processed foods, candy, cookies, cake, ice cream, etc.

No coffee, tea, cow's milk or alcohol

No relish, spices, vinegar, mustard, soy sauce, or ketchup

No oil or butter or fried food (except the 1 Tbsp. oil daily)

No dairy products, eggs, milk, cheese or yogurt

PHASE TWO: SAMPLE MEAL PLANNER

Upon arising, have some water or the *Lemon Drink.

Breakfast

An all-fruit meal is ideal in the warmer months or a warmer climate, if you are not diabetic or hypoglycemia. Have a handful of nuts or seeds for protein with your fruit. (I don't recommend eating a lot of fruit in the winter, since this can lower your body's resistance to colds. Try to eat foods in season as much as possible.)

Choose from:

One or two small pieces of fresh fruit: one apple, grapefruit, banana, orange, plums, strawberries, cherries, nectarine, peach, or pear. Fresh fruit is preferable over canned, cooked, or frozen fruit. Have some sunflower seeds, almonds, walnuts or cashews.

Optional:

Here is a special juice that is cleansing for the liver

Liver Cleanse Juice

6-8 carrots

1 apple

1 stalk celery

$^1/_4$ beet

Snack: Ten raw nuts or a handful of raw sunflower seeds

Lunch

Try to have a large vegetable dish, animal or vegetable protein and one-half to one serving of a complex carbohydrate.

Choose from:

1. Vegetable salad, grilled chicken strips (or vegetarian protein) and one slice of Whole-grain bread

2. Stir-fried vegetables, baked salmon (or tempeh or tofu), and one-half of a baked potato

3. Steamed vegetables, turkey breast (or tempeh or tofu), and one slice of bread or a baked yam

Dressing: Make an olive oil, lemon dressing. See the recipe section for healthy salad dressings.

Snack: Ten raw nuts or a handful of raw sunflower seeds

Dinner

Same as lunch. Try to have a large vegetable dish, animal or vegetable protein and one-half to one serving of a complex carbohydrate.

CONCLUSION:

Following Phase Two, go back to Phase One, gradually adding dairy and spices. Try to follow the Life Design Principles included in this book, and be sensitive to your body's needs for protein. Here are additional tips:

1. If you find that you are eating too many carbohydrates, then cut back by one serving every other day. If you aren't steadily losing weight when eating four carbohydrate servings per day, then cut back to three carbohydrate servings. This strategy has helped several of my clients eliminate carbohydrate cravings. Some even had to cut their servings to one or two carbohydrates a day. After they eliminate their cravings, and complete the Six week plan, they can go back to a higher number of carbohydrate servings.

2. If you overeat a meal or several times in a day, then on the next day, cut back on your portions at all meals.

3. If you can't seem to lose those last few pounds, then eat your normal foods on one day, and the next day, cut back your calories slightly. Then go back to your normal meals on the next day and so on. Follow this pattern for two or three weeks.

Don't be discouraged if you don't see immediate weight loss following any of these ideas. It has taken one to three months for many of my clients to really see a difference in their body's ability to burn fat. Give yourself time as you re-balance your body.

Recommended Supplements

- Digestive enzymes for the stomach
- Liver cleansing product
- One tablespoon flaxseed oil
- Psyllium powder and/or herbs for the colon
- Calcium lactate supplement (1,000 mg.)

See chapter 21 for recommended supplements and a summary of the supplements recommended throughout this book.

It's easy for me to eat healthy, cleansing foods. Cleansing, eating light, and occasional fasting helps me lose weight, and stay healthy and strong.

Chapter Twenty

Shopping: Where Is the Good Stuff?

Shopping in a supermarket can be an overwhelming experience! Bill, another client recently said, "I go to the grocery store with a conscious decision to read the labels and buy healthy foods. Thirty minutes later, I just give up and throw whatever I see in the basket! It's too overwhelming to read every label. Even then, you don't know what you're getting!"

Find Healthier Options

This is a common reaction! Americans are so accustomed to buying and eating processed foods that we find it awkward and even difficult to change. How can you quickly spot healthy foods among so many processed ones?

Throughout the years, I have accompanied clients as they shopped in their local grocery stores teaching them to sort through the thousands of packaged foods and make smarter selections. I recently did this with a client. We went through a grocery store, which is one of the national chain supermarkets. Come through the aisles with us and see what we found.

Fruits:

Here we are at the produce aisles looking at whole fresh fruits. Here's where you want to stock up! Fresh produce is packed with vitamins, minerals and enzymes, all vital for healthy weight loss. If you can, get up to 50 percent of fruits and vegetables in your eating plan.

It's best to eat fruits alone, in their raw, fresh state. Many people like to make a meal of a fruit salad, or eat them as snacks. Either way, most people need some protein for breakfast too, so add some raw nuts such as almonds or cashews (ten per day). Canned fruit has no enzymes and often is loaded with extra sugar, so frozen is preferred over canned. If you do use canned fruit, buy the fruit packed in light syrup, or with no added sugar.

Vegetables:

Also in the produce section, you find all the fresh vegetables. You can eat vegetables raw, lightly steamed, in a salad, baked or stir-fried, with a little bit of olive oil or butter. Herbal seasonings add some flavor.

As for salads, look for the dark-green leafy vegetables like Romaine and green leaf lettuce. Forget the iceberg lettuce; it contains little nutrition. Your local grocery store and health food store both carry ready-to-eat salad mixes.

Read a label or two on canned vegetables and you'll see that sugar is commonly added! Ditch the canned vegetables, and for convenience, get frozen vegetables. The trick here is to get them without all those extra fatty sauces, sugar or chemicals.

Fruits	Vegetables
• Apples	• Alfalfa sprouts
• Applesauce, unsweetened	• Artichokes
• Apricots	• Asparagus
• Bananas	• Bamboo shoots
• Berries:	• Beets/beet greens
Blackberry	• Bok choy
Blueberry	• Bell peppers
Boysenberry	• Broccoli
Cranberry	• Brussels sprouts
Elderberry	• Cabbage
Gooseberry	• Carrots
Raspberry	• Cauliflower
Strawberry	• Celery
• Cherries	• Corn on the cob
• Dates	• Cucumbers
• Figs: dried or fresh	• Endive
• Grapefruit	• Green beans
• Grapes: red or green	• Leeks
• Kiwi fruit	• Lettuce: red, green leaf
• Lemons	• Mushrooms
• Limes	• Onions: red, white
• Mandarin oranges	• Peppers: bell, cherry, red

Fruits

- Mango
- Melons:
    Cantaloupe
    Cassava
    Honeydew
    Watermelon
- Nectarines
- Oranges/Tangerines
- Papaya
- Passion fruit
- Peaches
- Pears
- Pineapple
- Plums
- Prunes
- Raisins
- Watermelon
- Fruit leather (100% fruit)

Vegetables

- Potatoes: red, white
- Radishes
- Romaine lettuce
- Snow peas
- Spaghetti squash
- Spinach
- Squashes
- Sugar snap peas
- Tomatoes
- Turnips
- Yams
- Watercress
- Zucchini

Salad Dressings:

Many people skip the French Fries, but they load their salads with hydrogenated salad dressings or mayonnaise. Check out the labels on many of the grocery salad dressings and you'll also find sugar or hydrogenated oils! Here are some healthy suggestions. You are allowed some fat in your diet. Use extra-virgin olive oil or flaxseed oil and lemon juice for your salads. Get a healthy (non-hydrogenated) salad dressing like Cardinis. Or go to your local health food store and buy a "healthy" fat-free salad dressing like some of these listed below.

- Tree of Life Low-fat dressings
- Spectrum Dressings (Low-fat Southwest Caesar, Honey Dijon)
- Annie's Naturals Salad Dressings
- Cardini's Salad Dressings
- Paul Newman's Own Salad Dressings
- Nasoya Nayonaise (Tofu salad dressing)

- Nasoya Vegi Dressings (in place of mayonnaise)
- Spectrum Canola mayonnaise
- Spectrum Lite Canola Mayonnaise
- Spectrum Vegetable Oils (Olive Oil, Canola, etc.)
- Hain Mayonnaise and oils
- Barlean's Fresh Express Flax Oil

Condiments:

When you pay close attention to the labels on the condiments aisle, you'll be amazed at how many condiments are packed with corn syrup, dextrin, monosodium glutamate (MSG), and sugar in many forms. It's almost impossible to find a spaghetti sauce without high fructose corn syrup and cottonseed oil! In your grocery store, Sutter Home and Classico are two companies who make tomato sauces without sugar or hydrogenated oils.

At the local health food store, look for the brand Enrico's or any of the other wonderful home-style cooked tomato sauces. Many of my clients prefer Bragg's Amino Acids in place of salt or soy sauce. Your health food store also has sugar-free condiments.

- Bernard Jensen's Vegetable broth and seasoning
- Bragg's Liquid Aminos
- Westbrae or Tree of Life Dijon mustard
- Westbrae Tamari soy sauce (low sodium)
- Eden soy sauce
- Sutter Home tomato sauce
- Classico tomato sauces (read labels; some varieties contain sugar)
- Enrico's spaghetti sauces and condiments
- Tree of Life spaghetti sauce
- Muir Glen spaghetti sauce
- Bragg's Apple cider vinegar, raw, unpasteurized
- Brown Rice vinegar (Spectrum Foods)
- San-J wheat-free Tamari
- Salsa
- Barbecue sauce
- Chili sauce

Jams and Jellies/Nut Butters:

After the condiments, we came to the section containing all the jams and jellies. My client and I read labels for almost twenty minutes before we found some jams and jellies without added sugar (high fructose corn syrup) and hydrogenated oils!

The best choices in your grocery store are Smucker's Simply Fruit and Polaner's All Fruit. They're sweetened simply with fruits and fruit juices. Below I've listed additional nut butters like those made with almonds, or sesame seeds. Children especially love the taste of natural almond butter! I've also added nonsweetened applesauce to the list since many of the varieties are loaded with sugar. Musselman's was the only one we could find in the grocery store that did not have added sugar. Your health food store will have more choices.

- Smucker's Natural Peanut Butter
- Smucker's Simply Fruit
- Arrowhead Mills Almond Butter, Peanut Butter, Cashew Butter, Sesame Tahini
- Apple Butter (unsweetened)
- Musselman's natural applesauce
- Polaner's jams
- Maranatha Nut Butters (Almond, Cashew, Macadamia Nut, Sunflower)

Breads:

Another overwhelming place is the bread aisle! My client and I looked at loaf after loaf before we found natural, whole grain breads. Two names to look for in your grocery stores are Orowheat and Earth Grains. Most health food stores carry Ezekiel Bread, which is a wonderful whole grain bread, based on a Bible recipe (Ezekiel 4:9). Look for sprouted, seven or ten-grain breads. In Tulsa, we are fortunate to have a Big Sky Bakery, which majors on whole grain baked goods. Another good choice are the nine-grain products at St. Louis Bread Company chains. Locally, your grocery store might carry variations like seven- or eleven-grain breads. If they're really made with whole grains, they're great! Here are some selections to look for:

- Orowheat Honey Whole Wheat, Oat Nut, Dark Rye and Seven Grain, whole-wheat Serenity Farms unyeasted and yeasted flat breads

- Shiloh Farms
- Earth Grains whole-wheat bread
- Wheat 'N Honey pocket Bread
- Ezekiel Bread
- Garden of Eatin breads
- Garden of Eatin Whole-wheat tortillas
- Garden of Eatin Whole-grain Pita bread
- Nature's Garden breads
- Nine-grain or sprouted bagels
- Bran muffins
- Whole-grain hamburger buns
- Rye crisp crackers
- Ak-Mak whole-wheat crackers
- Manna sprouted bread

Cereals and Whole Grains:

Judging from labels on common breakfast cereals, most kids in America are eating fat and sugar for breakfast! It's hard to find a cereal which contains lower than three to four grams of sugar per serving. Some are as high as thirteen grams (even in the health food store)! In your grocery store, those listed below are the best.

Avoid obvious high-fat cereals, which includes granola—a high-fat and high-sugar cereal! Not a good choice for weight loss. Brands to look for in the health food stores are Arrowhead Mills, Barbara's, Health Valley, Lundberg and New Morning. Whole grain waffles (Nutrigrain) are the best bet for waffles, but only on occasion because these are highly processed.

Besides oatmeal, brown rice is another cereal grain, much preferred over white rice, which has been refined. Brown rice comes in several varieties. Other options are quinoa, millet, or spelt. These are extremely nutritious grains; however, you may have to get used to their unusual flavors.

- Barbara's Shredded Spoonfuls
- Fiber One
- Kashi (not puffed)
- Kashi Good Friends (8 grams fiber per ¾ cup)
- Health Valley Muesli

- Roman Meal Cream of Rye
- Roman Meal Old Fashioned Oats
- All Bran Cereal
- Van's Whole Grain Waffles
- Barbara's Breakfast O's
- Shredded Wheat
- Slow Cooking Oatmeal
- Arrowhead Mills Bran or Corn Flakes
- Health Valley Oat Bran Flakes
- New Morning Honey Almond Oatios
- Uncle Sam's Cereal (with flax)
- Uncle Ben's Brown Rice
- Arrowhead Mills Short, long-grain brown rice
- Arrowhead Mills Wild Rice (Quick)
- Arrowhead Mills Quinoa (Whole grain)
- Arrowhead Mills Millet (Whole grain)
- Arrowhead Mills Spelt flakes

Pasta:

Most pastas are made with—you guessed it—refined white flour. What are better options? First, look for "colored" pasta, which are at least made with spinach, beets or other vegetables. Hodgson Mills is a common grocery store brand.

Pritikin, Deboles and Tree of Life makes delicious whole-wheat spaghetti and linguini. Wouldn't it be great if Italian restaurants used natural whole-grain pasta? Your health food store carries many varieties.

- Cleopatra's Kamut Pasta
- Pritikin Whole-Wheat Linguini
- Pritikin Whole-Wheat Spaghetti
- Debole's Pasta (many varieties, including whole-wheat)
- Tree of Life Pasta (not whole grain)
- Fantastic Pasta and Beans
- Vita Spelt Pasta
- Bionaturea Organic Pasta, Whole-Wheat

Proteins:

If you can get "organically grown" sources of meat, dairy or fish, then purchase those! Otherwise, select the leanest you can find and use red meat (preferably organically grown) in moderation.

I omit shellfish (lobster, crab, shrimp and oysters) because they are scavengers, and they are higher in saturated fat. Healthy, clean fish have fins and scales. Those are cleaning filters. Scavengers eat anything and everything, even toxic waste. This waste is stored in their bodies.

"Free range" means the animals were allowed to roam freely—not penned up. If they aren't exercising, they get fat, just like us! The leaner the meat, the better for you. Shelton is a manufacturer of organic chickens and turkeys. Shelton also makes wonderful canned Chicken Chili and Turkey Chili, found in your health food store. Other canned meat includes tuna fish packed in water, canned chicken and salmon.

Eggs and dairy organically grown are superior. Use small amounts of natural cheese.

Vegetarian proteins include beans, grains, and soy foods. Read labels on canned beans. Many of them contain sugar and lard! Look for just beans, water and salt. Heinz and Progresso are grocery store names. Arrowhead Mills, Health Valley, Hain, Westbrae, and Shelton are manufacturers of beans that you can find in the health food store.

Soy foods are becoming popular for their health benefits. Soy milk is wonderful, but look for a low-sugar one. Tempeh is made from beans and rice, and can be used in recipes in place of hamburger or bacon (See Lightlife product Fakin Bacon). Tofu is like a cheese and it has different styles. Firm tofu is good for a stir-fry, puddings and dips; and soft or silken tofu makes better protein drinks. Boca burgers are soy burgers that are flavored. Many of my clients really like them served on a whole wheat bun with mustard.

Recently, I've used Lightlife's Smart ground and found it to be an excellent substitute for red meat, without the saturated fat, but it contains twelve grams of protein. It's a soy-based, already prepared and flavored product. Just open and use where you would ground beef. Lightlife makes a variety of soy-based meat alternatives including Meatless Lightburgers, Smart Dogs, Fakin Bacon, and Smart Deli meatless fat-free slices. All of these taste great, are high in protein, contain no cholesterol, and barely any fat. You may even find these at your grocery store in the deli section.

Proteins:

Animal Sources:
Meat

- Buffalo meat
- Chicken breast (skinless)
- Cornish hen
- Ground turkey breast
- Ground chicken or turkey
- Canned chicken or white
- Venison

Vegetarian Sources
Beans: (Westbrae, Eden, Bearito, Heinz, Progresso)

- Aduki
- Black beans
- Black eyed peas
- Cannellini
- Fava
- Garbanzo
- Great Northern
- Kidney
- Lentils
- Lima
- Mung
- Navy
- Pinto
- Peas, green
- Red beans
- Split peas

Fish:

- Bass
- Bluefish
- Catfish
- Cod
- Flounder
- Haddock
- Halibut
- Mackerel
- Mahi mahi
- Ocean perch
- Orange roughy
- Red snapper
- Salmon
- Sardines

Soybean products:

- Tofu
- Tempeh
- Ready Ground Tofu
- Tofu burgers
- Boca Burgers
- Yves Veggie Burgers
- Lightlife Smart Dogs
- Lightlife Fakin' Bacon
- Lightlife Smart ground
- Lightlife Smart Deli
- Lightlife Meatless Lightburgers
- Baked, flavored Tofu
- Yves Veggie Tofu Wieners
- Pacific Soy Milk

- Snapper
- Trout
- Tuna
- Whitefish
- Tuna packed in water
- Canned salmon in water
- Canned sardines in water

- Soy Moo (Health Valley)
- Soylecious (Frozen Dessert)
- Soy Dream
- Eden Soy Milk
- Westbrae Soy Milk

Healthy Fats and Oils:

You probably know it's hard to find nonhydrogenated spreads. A great substitute for margarine is Spectrum Spread which is made from canola oil. Also, make your own "better butter" by mixing together equal parts of olive oil and butter. Use cold-pressed vegetable oils like olive oil and canola oil. You can find various types of olive oil at your grocery store. However, I recommend that you buy other oils, like canola oil or safflower at a health food store, since most grocery stores carry refined oils.

Vegetable sprays like Tyson's or Pam's pump spray are good. The following are healthier alternatives you may find at your health food store.

- Raw butter
- Spectrum Spread
- Bionaturea olive oil
- Spectrum cold pressed natural oils
- Spectrum cold-pressed, extra-virgin olive oil
- Barlean's Flaxseed oil
- Spectrum Cold-pressed sunflower, canola and sesame oil
- Avocados
- Nature's Cuisine all-natural olive oil spray
- Almonds, raw
- Arrowhead Mills Sunflower seeds
- Arrowhead Mills Sesame seeds
- Arrowhead Mills Flax seeds
- Pecans, raw
- Pistachio nuts, raw
- Walnuts, raw
- Cashews, raw
- Pumpkin seeds, raw

Dairy:

You'll notice I'm not a "got milk" advocate! In working with people over these years, we've seen that dairy is best eaten "pre-digested," as in yogurt, cottage cheese, buttermilk and kefir. You may not be familiar with kefir, but it's a delicious cultured food most often found like a drinkable milk with fruit added.

Eliminate obvious "processed" cheeses. Your best bets are natural cheeses, without added colorings. Use cheese very moderately. Let's say just one or two tablespoons in a topping to replace that whole cup of cheese.

- Organic Valley milk
- Alta Dena milk
- Alta Dena buttermilk
- Alta Dena Kefir
- Alta Dena Nonfat, plain yogurt (sweetened with juices)
- Chino Valley (free range)
- Alta Dena Low-fat or raw cottage cheese
- Tree of Life Low-fat or raw cottage cheese
- Eggs (organic, or Eggland's Best)
- Butter
- Acidophilus milk
- Buttermilk, low-fat
- Mozzarella, part skim
- Parmesan cheese
- Natural Farmer's cheese
- Romano Cheese
- Feta cheese

Miscellaneous for Cooking:

Your family will appreciate a few snacks, so why not stock up on some healthier ingredients for your special baking? Substituting whole grain pastry flour cup-for-cup for white flour works in most recipes. Your natural foods store has a variety of cookbooks to help you. The following is a list of various ingredients for cooking and baking.

- Body Ecology Stevia Powder
- Stevita Stevia powder

- Sucanat
- Mori-Nu Tofu Mates (Lemon, Vanilla and Chocolate pudding mixes)
- Wonderslim 100% caffeine free cocoa
- Rumford's Non aluminum baking powder
- Ener G egg replacer
- Wonderslim Egg and fat replacer
- Sucanat Organic (natural, raw) sugar
- Maple Syrup (pure)
- Arrowhead Mills Pancake mixes, whole grain
- Vanilla (pure)
- Bob's Red Mill Whole-wheat flour
- Bob's Red Mill Whole-wheat pastry flour
- Arrowhead Mills Whole-wheat flour
- Arrowhead Mills Whole-wheat pastry flour
- Powdered skim milk
- Real salt
- DeSauza's Solar sea salt
- Tree of Life maple syrup
- Shady Maple Farms maple syrup

Fast-Food Health Food:

One of the most common complaints I receive from my clients is "How can I make meals my family likes, like macaroni and cheese, but healthy?" Great question! Sheila, a friend and client, makes homemade lasagna using a healthy spaghetti sauce, whole-wheat lasagna noodles and healthy cheeses. A great idea. You'll find healthier packaged and frozen versions of these foods at your health food store. Amy's is a common brand. Look for:

- Tree of Life Easy Meals
- Taste Adventure's dry soups, chilis, and instant beans
- Whole grain burritos
- Pizza
- Lasagna
- American puree entrees
- Cedarland entrees

- Amy's entrees
- Lundberg Farms packaged meals
- Fantastic packaged meals and meals in a cup
- Health Valley soups, packaged meals and meals in a cup
- Fantastic Foods rice and beans
- Fantastic Foods tabouli
- Fantastic Foods burger mix
- Arrowhead Mills Quick brown rice
- Cascadian Farms frozen meals: Morrocan, Mediterranean, Cajun, Oriental
- Chow mein noodles
- Water chestnuts
- Bamboo shoots
- Canned pasta sauces
- Canned tomatoes and tomato sauce
- Imagine Foods Aseptic pack soups and sauces
- Pacific Organic Aseptic pack sauces and broths (dairy and non-dairy)

Healthy Beverages:

Going down the beverage aisle in the grocery store is another shocker! The majority of beverages were packed with sugar. Many so-called fruit juices are not real fruit juice, but rather fruit drinks. Look for 100 percent orange juice with no sugar added. Gatorade is just water sweetened with sugar and chemicals! Make these choices instead:

- Pure water
- Teecino herbal coffee
- Cafix, Pero, or Postum
- Chinese green tea
- Herbal teas: (Try a Celestial Seasonings Sampler pack)
  Chamomile
  Red Zinger
  Mint tea
  Rosehips
  Sleepy Time
  Wild Berry
  Peppermint

- Raja's cup (Antioxidant tea)
- Organic coffee (sparingly)
- Alta Dena Yogurt Drinkables (Yogurt drink)
- Perrier water
- Campbell's tomato juice
- Lemon water
- Gerolsteiner Mineral water
- Freshly squeezed fruit and vegetable juices
- R. W. Knudsen juices
- Mountain Sun Juices
- Eden soy milk
- Westbrae soy milk
- Soy Dream
- Soy Moo
- Kogee 100% organic coffee
- Kogee decaffeinated coffee
- C Hatfield's no-sugar coffee mix
- Naturally Almond (almond drink)

Healthy Snack Foods:

Sheila also told me her children were delighted when they tasted the "healthy" snacks available. Here are some suggestions for your next "snack attack!" Health Valley makes many types of low-fat, healthy snacks, cereal bars, granola bars and much more.

- Wasa Bread crackers
- Kavli all-natural, whole-grain Crispbread
- Garden of Eatin' Blue Chip corn chips
- Garden of Eatin' bean chips
- Health Valley nonfat granola bars
- Health Valley Fat-free cookies
- Pride O' the Farm Whole-wheat fig bars
- Heaven Scent lowfat cookies
- Frozen fruit bars
- Nonfat frozen yogurt (eat sparingly)
- Westbrae cookies
- Rye Crisp

- Tree of Life saltines
- Bearitos No-fat snacks
- Guiltless Gourmet baked chips
- Barbara's Fat-free fig bars
- Mori-Nu tofu mates
- Pamela's Shortbread Cookies

What I eat matters! Planning meals and shopping is a vital part of my weight loss strategy. If it's out of my sight, it's out of my mind. So I stock my refrigerator and cupboards with safe, healthy foods.

Chapter Twenty-One

Supplements: How Much Do I Need?

K aren came to my office in tears. Every one of her weight loss efforts failed. After consulting with Karen, I gave her an eating plan and recommended several nutritional supplements. "Why do I have to take supplements?" she asked. "Can't I lose weight just with food?"

If you were raised in the States or any where processed foods are available, then probably not. Changing your diet is vital. Regular exercise is vital. But it's hard to restore proper organ functioning and nutritional deficiencies with diet alone. Drinking freshly squeezed juices is one way that many people have cleansed and overcome nutritional deficiencies. Usually further supplements are required. I've found most people need additional support for their stomach, colon, liver, thyroid or adrenals, even when juicing and eating lots of fresh fruits and vegetables.

We Don't Live in a Perfect World

We should be able to eat healthy meals and never need to take extra supplements. That may have been true in this country one hundred years ago before our soils were depleted and before the processing of foods, but it's not true today. There are simply too many elements that can cause people to become mineral and vitamin deficient. There has never been a scientific study to prove that our typical American diet meets the requirements for all the vitamins, minerals and other nutrients required for optimal health.

Are We Healthy?

Just look at our health rating as a nation—dozens of other nations rank higher than us! Many Americans suffer from numerous nutritional deficiencies. The Surgeon General reported that six of the ten leading diseases are diet related. That means degenerative diseases are nutrient-deficient related.

Do I Need Supplements?

There are a certain number of vitamins, minerals, protein, and essential fats that you need every day. Essential means that your body needs them, but doesn't make them without food. There are two reasons why we really need to supplement our diets.

First, processed and refined foods don't contain enough vitamins and minerals to meet the RDA.

Second, our lifestyles and habits prevent us from processing fully the food we eat. For example, drinking coffee, tea, and eating certain spices can deplete your store of vitamins and minerals, especially the B vitamins and calcium. Taking laxatives, smoking, overcooking food, or eating processed foods also deplete your nutritional backup. Drugs, accidents and illness, oral contraceptives, and poor diet can all take their toll. Other reasons are poor digestion, stress, PMS, pregnancy, food allergies, fad diets, and drinking alcohol. Following workouts, athletes too may find that they lack essential vitamins and minerals for rebalancing the body.

Deficiencies Don't Happen Overnight

It may take months before vitamin or mineral deficiencies show up and when symptoms do occur (as in Chronic Fatigue), it takes an aggressive nutritional supplementation program to make up for these deficiencies.

Are All Supplements the Same?

Like my client, Bob, you stand at the supermarket or drugstore looking at all the supplements available and wonder, "What's the difference?" So you grab whatever and figure that will do. You may be like many of my clients who have a cabinet full of a variety of supplements and vitamins, but you still don't feel any better.

Whenever I have counseled anyone, I have asked my clients to bring in a list of the supplements they are taking, or the bottles themselves, so we can study the ingredients together. My clients often tell me they have taken some type of vitamin for a period of time and either it never worked or it worked at first and then stopped "working." Even supplements that I had been using seemed to lose their effectiveness after awhile. I was puzzled about this until I learned about the difference between various types of supplements: whole food, crystalline or synthetic vitamins.

What Are Natural Whole Food Supplements?

Natural supplements are whole foods with only the water and fiber removed. These are the most natural form of supplementing your diet. You can generally tell if a supplement is natural because the label will list the food sources from which these foods were obtained. A great example of natural whole food supplements sold through health professionals is Standard Process. These supplements are made from organically-grown whole foods and processed with low heat, so it doesn't destroy the enzymes. Examples of whole foods are wheat germ, brewer's yeast, and acerola cherries.

Just because the label says "natural," doesn't mean it is! Many supplements never break down! My greatest caution is against cheap, inexpensive off-brand, or mail order supplements. They often contain additives, food allergens, sugar, artificial food coloring, flavoring, shellac, chlorine, and other potentially hazardous chemicals. Many are not fresh. Not only are you wasting your money, but you could end up with problems like kidney stones from taking synthetic supplements.

Crystalline

Crystalline means it had a natural food as its original source but it was treated with various high-powered chemicals, solvents, heat, and distillations. Few enzymes remain.

Synthetic

Synthetic means the scientist has reconstructed the exact structure of the crystalline molecule by "putting together" the same molecules from other sources. As a vitamin, there is no difference between synthetic and crystalline. On the label for either, only the chemical name of the single vitamin is usually given. Both are heated and contain few enzymes.

Natural Compared to Synthetic

One of my peers, Juli Keene, C.N. told me about Standard Process supplements. When I switched from synthetic to natural supplements, my clients and I noticed a great difference! They reported feeling better within days. Their blood profiles improved consistently and dramatically.

One of my favorite multiple vitamins is Catalyn produced by Royal Lee in 1929 (Standard Process). Vitamins are catalysts in the body. Catalyn is the original catalyst, and it's ingredients and formula have remained unchanged for seventy years.

To fully understand the difference between types of supplements, just compare an orange to ascorbic acid (commonly known as vitamin C). The orange has the full vitamin C complex with all of the enzymes, coenzymes, antioxidants, trace elements, activators, and other unknown factors that cause the vitamin to work. Ascorbic acid is only one part of this once whole food! You can't take a complex apart and expect it to work the way God designed it. Once it has been separated, several components are missing. If your body already has the co-factors to recombine and process ascorbic acid, you could experience some improvement for a time. If you don't, the ascorbic acid won't benefit you. The symptoms you were trying to eliminate will return, and you could end up with a vitamin C deficiency!

Adding More Stress

Dr. Bruce West, in his publication, *Health Facts for the New Millennium,* explains the vital difference this way:

> Vitamins (such as vitamin B, C, and E) are complexes made up of a myriad of nutritional components. When you take one isolated synthetic fraction of this complex (perhaps ascorbic acid or alpha tocopherol), it's necessary for your body to assemble the entire nutritional complex from your existing nutritional stores in order for you to utilize the vitamin. If you do not have a sufficient nutritional store of the needed nutrients, the synthetic vitamin will simply fail to work. Even worse, when larger and larger doses of synthetics are ingested, you can actually cause nutritional deficiencies. How? Your body depletes stores of nutrients in an effort to make the synthetic fractions into whole vitamin complexes that can be used by your body.[1]

You Get What You Pay for

Synthetic vitamins are cheaper than natural supplements, since natural supplements involve growing whole food substances. However, I've found that a small amount of a vitamin in its whole-food form is much more effective, nutritionally, than a large amount of a synthetic one. I've listed a customer service number for Standard Process supplements in the Resources (Appendix J.) They can direct you to a health professional in your area. Otherwise, find a health food store that is likely to carry natural, food-based supplements. Generally, drugstores and grocery stores only carry synthetic vitamins.

Be a Smart Shopper

Remember, look for the names of whole foods on the label, rather than names of chemicals you cannot understand, spell, or pronounce! Make sure these supplements came from whole foods that were processed with low heat so as not to destroy the enzymes or the nutrition.

Another good way to tell if your vitamins are synthetic is to look at your urine. Synthetic vitamins, especially the B complex make your urine yellow. Don't waste your precious money on synthetic supplements which create expensive urine and may damage your health!

You Can Afford It!

When people first change their diets, they often make changes like adding a protein drink or nutritional food supplements. Adding more expense on top of a grocery-food budget can seem overwhelming. That's why I help people go through their diets and ditch all of the junk and nutrient-depleting foods. You know the ones I mean—potato chips, corn chips, doughnuts, coffee, and soda pops in all forms. You can save money just making that step.

Instead of spending money on coffee and a doughnut in the morning, why not use that money to have a protein drink! The money you save on junk foods can be well spent on a good food supplement. As a bonus, you won't be further depleting your body of vital nutrition! You'll feel better, have more energy, and look better when you eat wholesome foods.

Are Natural Supplements Safe?

The majority of the hundreds of clients I've counseled have improved their health dramatically by taking natural food supplements. Natural supplements that I am discussing are healthy, safe, food-based supplements. Synthetic, or man-made vitamins are not necessarily safe. Realize too that prescription and over-the-counter drugs kill between 100,000 and

200,000 people in the United States. Synthetic or man-made vitamins are toxic and certainly many adverse reactions are linked to them. Healthy supplements are health building not health destroying. I have never heard of a case where healthy supplements hurt anyone. If you are allergic to natural supplements, you probably have a toxic liver and/or kidneys.

What About Liquid Mineral Supplements?
Nature gives us natural, chelated minerals in plant foods such as vegetables. The plants take the inorganic minerals and convert them to a very available type of organic minerals that we can easily absorb. I have not seen any clinical evidence that liquid minerals from rocks are absorbable and I recommend my clients get their minerals from fruits and vegetables. If they supplement, I recommend whole-food, organically-grown supplements that are vacuum dried with low heat into tablets. I've found these to be far more effective than any other type of supplement.

How Much Do I Need?
I have been using whole food supplements for several years, and I've found that lower dosages of natural foods are more effective than high dosages of synthetic vitamins. My clients who are used to taking higher dosages are amazed at how well natural supplements work.

Most high-potency vitamin B pills are thiamine. Your body can only absorb 2-5 mgs. daily, yet most B vitamins contain 50 to 100 mg. Two problems come from taking synthetic vitamins. It can stress your body as you struggle to metabolize the chemicals. And secondly, these supplements are toxic. Excess B supplements made with thiamine are linked to the rise of sterility in this country.

Two things I recommend when taking supplements.

1. Buy them as natural as you can find.

2. Take digestive enzymes with them and drink lots of water.

Here is a general list of recommended supplements. Work with your health care provider for dosages. Additionally, you may want to supplement your diet with any of the recommended supplements listed in Chapters 3 to 11.

1. A plant-based digestive enzyme supplement that contains ample amounts of protease, lipase and amylase.

2. A natural-based multiple vitamin/mineral. Synthetic vitamins are toxic to the liver and create further stress.

3. An antioxidant (includes natural vitamins A, C, E and the mineral selenium).

4. Calcium/magnesium supplement or other bone building formula. Avoid calcium carbonate (such as Tums, and oyster shell supplements). A vegetable-based calcium is easily metabolized.

5. Many people who are overweight are deficient in the B complex vitamins, so vital for proper carbohydrate metabolism. This supplement often helps curb cravings, too.

6. Essential oils that contain essential fatty acids important in making prostaglandins for proper hormone function.

Below is a recap of the above. Note that the dosages here are general. Many natural supplements may have lower dosages than these, but are as effective.

Recommended Supplements

Multiple Vitamin/Mineral
Vitamin A: 5,000 mg.
Vitamin C: 500 mg.
Vitamin E: 400-600 I.U.
Selenium: 200 mcg.
Calcium: 1,000 mg.
Magnesium: 500 mg.
B complex: 25-50 mg.
1 Tbsp. flaxseed (or equivalent capsules)

Here is a recap of the supplements given in the "Nutritional Summary" sections throughout this book starting with chapter three.

Remember, it may be overwhelming to take everything listed. Start with an enzyme, or colon cleanse. Then, decide which section you want to work on.

Chapter Three: How's Your Tummy?

- Take digestive enzymes
- Follow food-combining principles
- Take a Betaine Hydrochloride (or HCl) supplement
- Take a daily apple cider vinegar drink

Chapter Four: Me, Constipated?

- Drink six to eight 8-oz. glasses of water a day
- Get regular exercise
- Eat a healthy diet
- Take a fiber supplement
- Eat cultured foods like yogurt, or take an acidophilus supplement
- Do a colon cleanse at least twice a year
- Consider taking colonics

Chapter Five: How's Your Liver?

- Drink the Lemon Drink
- Take digestive enzymes
- Juice carrots, beets and apples daily
- Take a B complex supplement daily
- Take liver support herb such as Milk Thistle
- Take 1 Tablespoon of flaxseed oil daily
- Take a lipotropic
- Take antioxidant supplements (vitamins A, C, E and the mineral selenium)
- Take a garlic supplement - 2 capsules three times daily

Chapter Six: Are You Revved Up or Burned Out?

- See a health professional about a natural thyroid hormone
- Take a kelp or natural iodine supplement
- Check your zinc and selenium
- Take a L'tyrosine supplement
- Take desiccated thyroid supplement
- Take the B complex
- Take antioxidant supplements

Chapter Seven: Are You Sneezy, Grumpy, and Dopey?

- Eliminate possible allergens
- Take digestive enzymes
- Eliminate stimulants like coffee and sugar.
- Supplement the diet with the antioxidant vitamins (A,C, E, and selenium), garlic, and essential fatty acids.
- Supplement your diet with Chromium GTF or L'glutamine if you are struggling with starch, sugar or alcohol cravings.

Chapter Eight: Sugar High Got You Low?

- Take Chromium GTF (200 mcg.)
- Take antioxidants: A, C, E and selenium
- Take the B complex supplements (25-50 mg.)
- Eat a high-fiber diet
- Take L'glutamine supplement (500 mg. on an empty stomach, only with your doctor's permission)

Chapter Nine: Is Candida Driving You Crazy?

- Take a yeast killer
- Take digestive enzymes
- Take yogurt or acidophilus supplements
- Take antioxidants
- Take a garlic supplement

Chapter Ten: I'd Die for a Twinkie!

- Take digestive enzymes
- Cleanse the colon
- Support the liver
- Take a fiber drink
- Take magnesium for chocolate cravings
- Take the B vitamin complex
- Eat balanced meals

- For sugar cravings, suspect allergies, low-blood sugar, Candida, or low thyroid (See Chapters 7, 8, 9 or 10, respectively.)
- Take a protein drink, or an amino acid supplement. Or consider taking 5HTP, L'glutamine, L'tyrosine with your doctor's permission, since these amino acids should not be taken if you are taking any medications. Additionally, you should not take these isolated aminos at the same time. I would recommend the L'tyrosine in the morning, L'glutamine at lunch and the 5HTP at night. Your doctor can test your amino acid levels with a blood plasma test.

Chapter Eleven: Are You Wacky for a Week?

- Get fiber in your diet
- Eat soy foods
- Take a calcium/magnesium supplement for painful periods.
- Take organic iodine for hot flashes
- Take flaxseed oil or Evening primrose oil for painful breasts. (See Chapter 14 on good fats.)
- For chocolate cravings, take 200 mg. of magnesium
- For sugar cravings, use the progesterone cream, take Chromium GTF, or take the amino acid L'glutamine. (Take amino acid supplements only with your doctor's permission.)
- For depression, eliminate sugar and stimulants, increase your protein and consider taking 5HTP. (See chapter 10 on cravings.)

I don't mind getting and taking natural food supplements. I'm not leaving my health or weight loss efforts to chance. I support my body with great nutrition. I'm more valuable to people and God when I'm healthy!

Summary of Motivational Statements

Introduction: *Everyone can win over weight! I can and will lose weight safely. Forget the past—it's a new day!*

Chapter One: *I don't need to diet any more. I can eat the right foods to make me healthy. I'm ready to get healthy and lose weight safely.*

Chapter Two: *I no longer need to stay the way I am. Things seen are about to change!*

Chapter Three: *Now I know how to eat to keep my tummy well. I love the foods that are good for me. Indigestion, heartburn and sluggish metabolism are now a thing of the past.*

Chapter Four: *I love how good I feel when my bloodstream and colon are cleansed and I eat healthy foods. It's worth the time it takes to cleanse my body!*

Chapter Five: *What I eat matters. I now choose to eat the right portions that are right for me. I eat when I'm hungry and stop when I'm full. I no longer want to overeat. I love how good I feel when I support my liver.*

Chapter Six: *I get the energy I need from good healthy foods, and not from dangerous pills. My body burns fat perfectly. I eat the right foods to support my thyroid.*

Chapter Seven: *I no longer have to drag myself around. I can eat foods which give me energy. I know which foods make me tired and it's easy to eliminate them and eat healthier foods.*

Chapter Eight: *Now that I know that refined white sugar makes me fat, it's easy for me to give it up. I love the taste of natural sugar found in dried and fresh fruits. I love how good I feel when I eat right!*

Chapter Nine: Simple, healthy foods are the best. I love to eat vegetables and good quality protein. This way of eating is easy. I love how good I feel when my body works properly.

Chapter Ten: I only eat the foods I need when I am really hungry. I can and do resist junk foods. I'm breaking the craving/binge cycle. Cravings are a thing of the past because I eat balanced meals.

Chapter Eleven: My hormones are balanced and my body works perfectly, as it was designed to work. I eat healthy foods to support my body. PMS, water retention, and cravings are gone. I am happy and healthy.

Chapter Twelve: It's easy for me to give up sugar. I love natural fruits and natural sweets. I have self-control. Sugar has no more power over me.

Chapter Thirteen: I love the taste of natural whole grains and whole grain products. Refined snacks don't even taste good to me anymore. I love how good I feel eating healthy foods!

Chapter Fourteen: I am no longer interested in eating fat-storing, artery-clogging, sickness-producing foods. I love wholesome, natural foods that help me burn fat!

Chapter Fifteen: I crave good protein, not greasy hamburgers. It's easy for me to eat the right kind and amount of healthy proteins for my body.

Chapter Sixteen: I choose to eliminate caffeine from my diet. I can wean myself off caffeine safely. It's not a hard thing. I feel great when I drink healthy beverages. Even water never tasted so good!

Chapter Seventeen: It's easy to change my diet! I will achieve my weight-loss goals if I don't give up. I love exercise. It's easy to lose weight when I do it right!

Chapter Eighteen: I love designing my life so I can eat well and lose weight safely. I take responsibility for what I eat. I love how great I feel when I eat healthy foods.

Chapter Nineteen: It's easy for me to eat healthy, cleansing foods. Cleansing, eating light, and occasional fasting helps me lose weight, and stay healthy and strong.

Chapter Twenty: *What I eat matters! Planning meals and shopping is a vital part of my weight loss strategy. If it's out of my sight, it's out of my mind. So I stock my refrigerator and cupboards with safe, healthy foods.*

Chapter Twenty-One: *I don't mind getting and taking natural food supplements. I'm not leaving my health or weight loss efforts to chance. I support my body with great nutrition. I'm more valuable to people and God when I'm healthy!*

Benefits of Apple Cider Vinegar

Apple Cider Vinegar helps:

- maintain a youthful vibrant body
- fight germs and bacteria naturally
- retard the onset of old age
- regulate calcium metabolism
- keep blood the right consistency
- regulate menstruation for women
- normalize the urine
- digestion and assimilation
- relieve sore joints, and cleans out toxins
- sinus and asthma sufferers to breathe easier
- maintain healthy skin
- prevent itching scalp, dry hair, baldness and banishes dandruff
- fight arthritis and removes toxins and crystals from joints, tissues and organs
- control and normalize weight[1]

Taken from *Apple Cider Vinegar* by Paul C. Bragg. Reprinted with permission.

Sodium Tips

W e need only 1-2 tsp. of salt daily. Many Americans consume five to twenty-five times more sodium than they need. But it's not always obvious to spot, and it all adds up. One teaspoon of salt equals about 2,000 mg. of sodium. Here are some tips for lowering your sodium intake.

- Replace the salt and pepper shakers with kelp and cayenne pepper or some other healthy herbs.
- Sea salt, herb salts, sesame salt, and natural soy sauce are good substitutes. Sea salt contains natural minerals that have not been refined out. Mrs. Dash is a good substitute for salt.
- When buying frozen entrees, look for the ones that contain between 800 and 1,000 mg. of salt. See Appendix E on Label Reading for more help. (Your health food store contains herbs, spices, and other low-salt condiments, including sea salt.)

Limit commercially-prepared condiments which are full of sodium:

Onion salt	Soy sauce
Celery salt	Steak sauce
Garlic salt	Barbeque sauce
Seasoned salt	Catsup
Meat tenderizer	Mustard
Bouillon	Worcestershire sauce
Baking powder	Salad dressings
Baking soda	Pickles
Monosodium Glutamate	Chili sauce

Sodium-containing ingredients you will want to eliminate or reduce are:

Baking powder
Baking soda
Monosodium glutamate
Sodium benzoate
Sodium caseinate
Sodium citrate
Sodium phosphate
Sodium proportionate
Sodium saccharin

Source: US Dietary Guidelines Bulletin 232-6

Glycemic Index

Low Glycemic Desirable Foods	Med. Glycemic Moderately Desirable	High Glycemic Least Desirable
Beans:		
Lentils	Pinto beans	
Black-eyed peas	Kidney beans	
Lima beans	Baked beans	
Chick peas	Chick peas, canned	
Navy beans	Garbanzo beans	
Butter beans	Lentils, canned	
Soy beans		
Tempeh		
Tofu		
Soy Burgers		
Vegetables:		
Tomatoes	Yams	Boiled white potatoes
Green peas	Frozen peas	Instant mashed potatoes
Artichoke	Beets	Instant potato
Broccoli		Microwaved potato
Asparagus		
Brussel sprouts		
Cauliflower		
Cucumber		
Celery		
Cabbage		
Green peppers		
Mushrooms		
Onions		
Radish		

Low Glycemic Desirable Foods	Med. Glycemic Moderately Desirable	High Glycemic Least Desirable
Grain, Cereals, and Breads:		
Oat Bran Cereals	Bran Chex	Instant cereals
All Bran	Grape Nuts	Flaked cereals
Slow-cooking oatmeal	Cream of Wheat	English muffins
Uncle Sam's Cereal	Museli	White flour doughnuts
Fiber One	Shredded Wheat	White breads
Oat Bran bread	Wasa Bread	Corn breads
Pumpernickel bread	Brown rice	Glutinous rice
Whole-grain rye bread	Instant oat cereal	Instant white rice
Protein-enriched	Ezekiel 4:9 bread	French bread
Spaghetti	Melba Toast	White bagel
Rice bran	Sprouted wheat bread	White pasta
Cooked bulgar	Shiloh Farms bread	White waffles and pancakes
Fruits:		
Cherries	Kiwi fruit	Banana, ripe
Grapefruit	Apple juice	Raisins, dried
Peaches	Applesauce	Mango
Plums	Orange	Pineapple
Pears	Orange juice	Fruit juice (sugar
Grapes	Prunes	sweetened)
Apples		
Snacks:		
Peanuts	Rye crispbread	Potato chips
Graham crackers	Microwave popcorn	Rice cakes
Almonds	Stone-ground	Oatmeal cookies
Walnuts	Wheat Thins	Sugar-sweetened cookies

How to Read a Food Label

When you are touring a country, you will always find it easier with a road map. The same applies as you weave your way up and down your local grocery store aisles. You need a guide. Nutritional companies are required to follow the labeling guidelines set by the US government.

The following information is taken from the U.S. Publication, *"How to Read The New Food Label."*

FATS

Fat-free or no fat:	Less than .5 grams of fat per serving
Low-fat:	Three grams of fat (or less) per serving
Low-saturated fat:	One gram or less per serving
Reduced or less fat:	No more than half the fat than the regular product
Reduced or less saturated fat:	At least 25% less per serving than the regular food

---

MEATS

Lean:	Less than 10 grams of fat, less than 4 grams of saturated fat, and less than 95 milligrams of cholesterol per serving
Extra lean:	Fewer than 5 grams of fat, less than 2 grams of saturated fat, and less than 95 milligrams of cholesterol per serving

---

SUGAR

Sugar-free:	Less than .5 grams per serving
Reduced sugar:	At least 25 percent less sugar per serving than the comparison food

No added sugar,
without added sugar,
no sugar added: No sugar added during processing

CALORIES
Calorie-free: Less than 5 calories per serving
Low-calorie: Less than 40 calories per serving
Reduced or fewer
   calories: At least 25 percent fewer calories per
                    serving than the regular food

CHOLESTEROL
Cholesterol free: Less than 2 milligrams of cholesterol and 2
                    grams or less of saturated fat per serving
Low cholesterol: 20 milligrams or less per serving
Reduced or less
   cholesterol: At least 25 percent less and 2 grams or less of
                    saturated fat per serving than the regular food

SODIUM
Sodium-free/salt free: Less than 5 mg. per serving
Low-sodium: Less than 140 mg. per serving
Very low sodium: Less than 35 mg. sodium per serving
Reduced sodium: At least 25 percent less than
                    comparison food

FIBER
High-fiber: 5 grams or more per serving
Good source of fiber: 2.5 grams to 4.9 grams per serving
More or added fiber: At least 2.5 grams more per serving
                    than the comparison food

LIGHT OR LITE
Light or lite: One-third less calories or no more than one-
                    half the fat of the higher-calorie, higher-fat
                    version, or no more than one-half the sodium
                    of the higher sodium version.

Source: "How To Read The New Food Label," Food and Drug Administration, FDA 93-2260.

Fat Formulas and Fats

Whenpeople begin to understand that "good" fat burns fat, it's easy to over do it. One tablespoon of cold-pressed olive oil has 13 grams of fat. While it's a good fat, too much fat can put you well over your 36 grams, or daily fat allotment in one meal! But I do recommend that you have at least a tablespoon a day. You can put it on your whole grain cereal, or in a salad dressing, or take it as a supplement.

FAT FORMULAS

1. Figuring the Number of Fat Grams in Your Diet

a. First, count up the number of calories in your daily intake. Let's say you eat 1500 calories and you want to stay within 30% of calories from fat.

b. Multiply 1500 (total calories) times 30% (percentage of fat) equals 450 calories from fat.

c. Divide 450 (the calories from fat) by 9 to determine how many grams of fat you should eat. In this case, it's 50.

This means if you eat 1500 calories, and you want to stay with 30% calories from fat, then eat no more than 50 grams of fat daily.

2. Figuring the Percentage of Fat in Your Diet

a. Take an average of your total calories and fat grams per day. Let's say you average 1500 calories per day and you average 60 grams of fat.

b. Multiply your grams of fat (60) times 9 (calories per gram) = 540 calories.

c. Divide the calories (540) by 1500 (total calories) = 36% of your calories is from fat.

---

3. Figuring the Percentage of Calories from Fat in Your Food

Let's say our product has 200 total calories and 8 grams of fat:

a. Find the total number of total calories on the food label - 200.
b. Find the total number of fat grams per serving on the food label - 8.
c. Multiply the number of fat grams (8) times 9 equals 72.
d. Divide that figure (72) by the total number of calories (200) equals 36% of calories are from fat.

KINDS OF FATS

1. Monosaturated Fats:

Best all purpose vegetable oils
Sources: olive oil, canola oil, peanut oil, avocados, peanuts, cashews, almonds
What they do:
Increase "good" HDL cholesterol
Decrease "bad" cholesterol

2. Polyunsaturated Fats:
(Including Essential Fatty Acids)

These oils include high amounts of essential fatty acids (EFAs), Omega 3 (linolenic) and Omega 6 (linoleic) oils from both animal or vegetable sources.

Sources: All other unrefined vegetable oils such as flaxseed, sesame, corn, cod liver, safflower, sunflower, cottonseed, walnut and primrose oils, sunflower and flax seeds. Also cold-water fish like salmon and mackerel, herring, cod, sardines and tuna.

What they do:
Increase "good" cholesterol
Decrease "bad" cholesterol
Decrease triglycerides
Reduce tendency to form blood clots in arteries

3. Saturated Fats:

Fats high in cholesterol mostly found in fats of animal origin. This includes oils usually solid at room temperature, hydrogenated fats found in hydrogenated margarines, lard, shortenings, and processed peanut butter, commercially-baked good and most fast food.

Sources: meat, fish, bacon, pork, ham, chicken, eggs, whole milk, cream, cheese, cream cheese, butter, coconut, coconut oil, cocoa butter, palm oils, ice cream and chocolate.

What they do:

Raise "bad" cholesterol or LDL

Lower "good" cholesterol or HDL

Contribute to heart disease and cancer

4. Trans Fats:

Fats that have been damaged by high heat.

Sources: These are found in most fast foods, margarine, shortening, processed baked goods (cookies, cakes and taco shells) with hydrogenated oils, all fried foods.

What they do:

Increase "bad" cholesterol

Lower "good" cholesterol

Can cause free radicals and cancer

Can cause premature aging

Getting Slim While Eating Out

Many of my clients faithfully eat healthy at home but lose direction when they eat out. They think, "I can eat well at home, but in a restaurant? No way!" There is a way. Let's look at general restaurant tips, eating fast food, and what to order at your favorite ethnic restaurant.

GENERAL RESTAURANT TIPS

Take your enzymes!

Carry a small container of enzymes in your purse or pocket so you will always have them with you. Just recently, my friend Jamie's mother had a stomachache after dinner. Her stomachache left immediately after Jamie gave her digestive enzymes.

Order Lemon water

Order water with lemon wedges on the side, to further aid the digestion process. (See chapter 4.) Rather than use white sugar or those "pink and blue" packets, use the "brown packets"—sugar in the raw. Better still, carry Stevia. I use it to sweeten lemon water, which makes a nice lemonade-type drink, or I use it to sweeten herbal tea. You can buy packets of stevia at your health food store or the sources found in Appendix J.

Have it Your Way!

You have a choice! You have a right to ask questions, or order food how you want it. For example, at a Chinese restaurant you can request food without MSG added. At a French restaurant, you can order fish or chicken grilled, not fried. Or, order a salad with dressing on the side and use their dressing sparingly.

Don't Eat it All Just Because You Can

Skip the all-you-can-eat buffets. You wind up eating *all* you can eat. It's great that you can serve yourself, but the fat grams add up fast.

The Skinny on Salad Bars

Wonder why we can still gain weight in spite of the popularity of salad bars? I've seen people make a great salad with vegetables like carrots, cucumbers, broccoli, mushrooms, green peas, and tomato—and then dump lots of high-fat salad dressing on top! Here are better suggestions.

- Just have a taste of salad dressing or any salads prepared with mayonnaise (coleslaw, potato salad, or macaroni salad).
- Try garbanzo beans, kidney beans, and turkey or chicken breast.
- Try nonfat yogurt, ask for low-fat salad dressing, or vinegar and olive oil dressing. Or bring your own.
- Skip the cheese, fried noodles, olives, and roasted, salted seeds.

Pick a Healthy Breakfast

Oatmeal or whole grain dry cereals with skim milk
Fresh fruit or fruit salads
Whole wheat toast or whole grain English muffins
Omelets with vegetables
Low-fat yogurt with fresh fruit and granola
Herbal tea
Poached eggs with whole grain toast

Skip the Appetizers

Don't eat before you eat! Wherever you eat, skip the bread and butter, chips and dip. Fill up on nutrient-dense foods such as chicken and vegetables.

Don't Eat Too Much

Most restaurant meals are too big. Just because it's sitting on your plate doesn't mean it has to go in your tummy. Split a dinner with a friend. Or, take some home for tomorrow's lunch.

Don't Drink!

Drinking alcohol puts fat on your liver and your body. All liquid sugar drinks are empty calories that deplete your vitamin and minerals.

Order Smart

Order entrees prepared in a low-fat way: broiled, steamed, poached, roasted, baked, grilled, or stir-fried. Try grilled or roast turkey, broiled fish, steamed vegetables, and lean meats. Order broiled chicken, chicken breast, or turkey sandwiches and leave off the cheese.

Try low-fat, whole-grain breads, mustard, lots of vegetables and lean meats.

Choose vegetable, tomato-based, or bean soups rather than creamed or cheese soups. Avoid casseroles.

Order a main course of vegetable, a side salad, and chicken appetizers.

For dessert, try fruit, low-fat frozen yogurt, sorbet, or angel food cake.

Avoid Artery-Clogging Fat

Here's the fat you want to avoid:
- Fried chicken, deep-fried foods, fried onion rings
- French fries, creamy sauces and dressings
- Pizza, sandwiches made with fatty meats like bologna, pastrami, sausage, and luncheon meat
- Chips and nachos

WHAT ABOUT FAST FOOD?

Ever wonder what to choose when you're in a rush and the only thing you can grab is "fast food?" Here are some tips and better choices:

Drink water instead of high-sugar beverages. If you are ordering fast food, order a small green salad with dressing on the side.

Grilled or roasted chicken sandwiches are one of your best choices.

Stick with plain burgers, baked potatoes, mashed potatoes, or corn on the cob.

Salad bar items to choose: greens, cottage cheese, vegetables without dressing, beans, and fruits.

Try roast turkey, roast chicken, and broiled fish.

Order sub sandwiches on wheat bread, with turkey or chicken and fresh vegetables. Omit the mayonnaise; try mustard instead.

Grilled chicken breast sandwiches, best on whole wheat bun*

Chicken salad with low-fat dressings or oil and vinegar dressing

(*Ask for a wheat bun if it's not on the menu.)

Skip:

French fries, onion rings and all fried foods

Avoid cheeseburgers and fried chicken

Also avoid pizzas, cheese sauces, creamy salad dressings, gravies, and coleslaw

Best Fast Food Choices

Wendy's: Grilled Chicken sandwich or pita pockets

McDonald's: McGrilled Chicken sandwich

Dairy Queen: Grilled Chicken sandwich

Arby's: Light Chicken or Turkey Deluxe sandwich

Taco Bell: Light Taco, Light Soft Taco, Light Taco salad without chips

SPECIALTY RESTAURANTS

American

Order grilled, steamed or baked lean meats (such as chicken or fish)

Choose salads with lean meats, all vegetables

Use salad dressing on the side, and dip with your fork before each bite, or ask for lemon juice, vinegar and seasonings

Look for whole-grain breads, non-creamy soups, whole-bean soups, baked potatoes, or better yet, baked yams

Skip:

Avoid french fries, gravies and sauces, fried chicken, potato skins, and fatty toppings

Mexican

Order Spanish rice, rice and bean dishes, gazpacho, or black-bean soup

Choose a taco salad, vegetable burrito, refried beans (without lard), chicken fajitas, chicken tacos

Order tostadas, burritos or enchiladas made with beans or chicken, rice, black beans, salsa, and steamed corn tortillas

Get guacamole or sliced avocado on the side

Order chicken soft tacos with little cheese

Order extra lettuce and tomato on the side for nutritional value without fat

Skip:

Flour tortillas (ask for whole grain tortillas if available)

Burritos, tostadas, tacos, and enchiladas made with beef, cheese and sausage

Nachos, con queso, fried tortilla chips, refried beans and corn tamales (both made with lard)

Hold the sour cream

Italian

Order a vegetable salad or plain pasta and broiled fish or chicken

Try pasta with red sauce, marinara sauce, or tomato-based sauces

Order clear white sauces, not creamy white sauces

Order lean meats

Try pasta primavera, minestrone soup, grilled chicken cacciatore, and chicken or veal picatta

Italian Ice is a fat-free dessert, but high in sugar, so only order a small portion if you can handle it.

Skip:

Pesto and cream sauces, and avoid deep-fried dishes, sausages, and salami

Cheesecake is high calorie and high fat

Avoid cheese-filled pasta, sausage dishes, cream and butter sauces, beef ravioli and lasagna

Chinese

Oriental food is not necessarily low fat! Ordering the wrong types of foods can cause you to eat as much fat as Mexican food.

I suggest that you go for lower-salt foods. A plus would be real buckwheat (soba) noodles.

If available, order brown rice rather than white rice

Ask for steamed rather than fried rice

Order steamed, stir fried, or boiled chicken and fish dishes that include vegetables and rice

Order clear soups, bean curd, and vegetable dishes

Most soups are okay unless you know they are made with oil

Skip:

Ask ahead and avoid foods made with monosodium glutamate (MSG*)

Avoid deep-fried egg rolls, fried noodles, and deep-fried dishes such as fried dumplings and fried wontons

(*MSG is an additive that makes some people nauseous. It has been known to adversely affect the nervous system.)

French

Try steamed or grilled fish or chicken breast or broiled lean meat

Order dishes prepared with wine sauces rather than butter or cream sauces

Choose seafood, poached fish, chicken in wine sauce, and steamed vegetables.

Choose fresh fruits, and cheese, and sorbet for dessert

Skip:

Avoid au gratin dishes made with cheese, cream sauces, butter sauces, blue cheese, or bernaise sauce (all made with eggs, butter, or cheese)

Avoid rich pastries

Japanese

Order grilled fish or chicken teriyaki, sukiyaki, stir-fried vegetables and broth-based soups

Order noodle soups and broth, bean sprouts and tofu

Also try miso or bean soups, udon noodles, steamed rice and rice noodles

Skip:

Avoid fried foods such as tempuras, fried chicken and fried pork

Avoid raw fish

Greek

Order shish kabob, grilled fish, grilled chicken, yogurt and cucumber dishes, rice pilaf and salads

Also try legumes, bean soups or lentil soup, eggplants, lentil soup, and grape leaves

Skip:

Deep fried dishes, creamy dishes, anchovies and baklava

Savvy Substitutions

INGREDIENT	SUBSTITUTE
Baking chocolate	Carob (one square) 3 Tbsp. carob plus 2 Tbsp. liquid or 3 Tbsp. powder plus 2 Tbsp. water
Baking powder	Aluminum-free baking powder
Biscuit mixes	Whole-grain mixes
Bouillon, beef or chicken	Vegetable broth, tamari, miso
Breads, muffins, pasta, etc.	Whole-grain breads, muffins, pasta, etc.
Canned fruit and vegetables	Fresh or frozen fruits and vegetables
Cheeses, processed	Tofu soy cheeses, yogurt cheese, almond cheese
Cereals, processed	Whole-grain cereals
Chips, processed, salted	Low-salt, low-fat, baked potato and corn chips
Cocoa	Carob powder (see above)
Coffee	Herbal teas
Condiments	Spices, low-salt condiments without sugar or extra salt or preservatives
Cornstarch	Arrowroot powder
Cottage cheese	Tofu
Distilled vinegar	Raw, unpasteurized vinegar or lemon juice

INGREDIENT	SUBSTITUTE
Ground beef	Tofu, miso, ground nuts, legumes, soy meatless ground, tempeh
Eggs, egg whites	Egg replacer, tofu
Flour, white, cake	Whole-wheat flour, oat flour, brown rice flour
Hydrogenated fats	Better butter (one part butter, one part olive oil)
Margarine, shortening	Cold-pressed, unrefined oils (olive, canola, sunflower, safflower)
Milk	Rice milk soy milk, almond milk
Pasta, spaghetti	Whole-wheat spaghetti, corn pasta, or rice pasta
Peanut butter, hydrogenated	Unhydrogenated peanut butter, sesame butter, almond butter, cashew butter, pistachio butter
Rice, white	Brown rice, buckwheat, amaranth, spelt, barley, millet, corn, oats, kamut
Salt, refined	Sea salt, Vegit, Spike, herbal seasoning, Mrs. Dash, or Tamari soy sauce
Sour cream	Blended tofu
Soy sauce	Natural tamari soy sauce
Spreads, jams, jellies	Unsweetened fruit spreads
Sugar	Honey, molasses, barley malt, brown rice syrup, Sucanat, date sugar, maple sugar, Stevia
Yogurt, commercial	Naturally fermented with live cultures
Whipped cream	Tofu whipped cream

Fat-Burning Recipes

T hese are recipes that I have developed and used in cooking classes for several years. They are taken from my forthcoming cookbook.

BEVERAGES

Lemon Drink

>1 cup water
>juice of one lemon
>**Optional:** 1 teaspoon honey, maple syrup, or dash Stevia

Drink hot or cold, but don't boil the lemon juice; add the lemon juice after heating the water.

Variation: 2 teaspoons of apple cider vinegar in 1 cup water with 1 teaspoon honey

Healthy Lemonade

>1 cup lemon juice (juice from 3-4 lemons)
>1 tablespoon honey or a few drops of Stevia liquid or powder
>5-6 cups of water
>ice

Blend ingredients well and serve cold.

Optional: A classic drink uses a dash of cayenne red pepper and raw maple syrup to stimulate digestion.

Protein Drink

> One scoop of protein powder*
> 1 cup of water or soy milk
> 1 tablespoon flaxseed oil
> Fruits as desired (banana, mango, pineapple, etc.)
> Crushed ice

Put everything in a blender and blend for a minute. (*You can purchase protein powders at your local health food store.)

Protein Drink Smoothie

Smoothies are quick, delicious, require few ingredients and always taste great! These protein drinks can be made with fruit, yogurt, milk, soy milk, almond milk or tofu. If you use tofu in place of yogurt, be sure to get one that is a "silken" variety. Make just enough for your meal because smoothies lose their punch if they sit too long.

> $1/2$ cup sliced fruit of choice
> 1 tablespoon honey or dash of Stevia powder
> $1/4$ teaspoon vanilla
> $1^1/2$ cups non-fat yogurt or silken tofu or 1 cup soy milk
> **Optional:** crushed ice. Add $1/2$ teaspoon cinnamon for additional flavor.

Blend all ingredients until creamy. Serve cold.

SALAD DRESSINGS

Basic Italian Dressing

A simple yet elegant Italian dressing.

> $1/4$ cup extra virgin olive oil
> $1/4$ cup lemon juice
> 1 clove garlic, minced
> dash sea salt
> **Optional:** 1 teaspoon each: marjoram, oregano and basil

Blend together and pour over a green salad.

No-oil Italian Dressing

It's possible to make a salad dressing without any fat or oil. Just use more herbs and vinegar. Here's a good no-fat dressing.

> $^1/_4$ cup lemon juice
> $^1/_4$ cup apple cider vinegar
> $^1/_4$ cup apple juice
> $^1/_2$ teaspoon each: oregano, garlic powder, rosemary, basil, sage and onion

Tofu Dijon Dressing

Tofu makes a creamy, rich dressing. Here's a nice tofu dressing that can be used as a dip, too.

> 16 ounces firm tofu
> 2 tablespoons vinegar
> 1 tablespoon Dijon mustard
> 1 tablespoon olive oil
> 1 teaspoon lemon juice
> 1 clove garlic, minced
> $^1/_4$ cup water

Combine in a blender and blend at low speed. This will last about a week in the refrigerator.

SALADS

Classic Mixed Green Salad

Here's a classic green salad, perfect for a lunch or dinner salad.

> 1 head chopped Green leaf lettuce
> 1 head chopped Romaine lettuce
> 3-4 shredded carrots
> 1 red pepper, sliced
> Other favorite salad vegetables

Dressing: Make your own from a good quality vegetable oil like olive oil or flaxseed oil, or buy a salad dressing that does not contain hydrogenated oils like Spectrum or Arrowhead Mills (found at specialty shops or health food stores). Another idea is to use avocado or salsa for a salad dressing.

Dijon Tofu "Eggless" Salad

This is one of the few places where I use raw tofu. In this salad, the tofu is crumbled finely with your hands and then well flavored with the dressing which contains Dijon mustard. The colored vegetables make a pretty as well as crunchy salad. It's nice served on salad lettuce leaves, too. Some people have never eaten tofu and are surprised at how good the salad tasted. If you don't have red pepper, try substituting tomatoes or radishes.

> 8 ounces firm tofu, drained and crumbled
> 1/4 cup leeks or green onions, chopped fine
> 1 clove garlic, minced
> 2 stalks celery, chopped fine
> 1/4 cup green pepper, chopped fine
> 1/4 cup red pepper or radishes, chopped fine
> 1/4 cup fresh parsley, minced

Dressing:

> 1/4 cup Dijon mustard
> 2 tablespoons olive oil
> 2 tablespoons red wine vinegar or apple cider vinegar
> dash salt and cayenne

Crumble tofu and combine with chopped vegetables in a salad bowl. Mix Dijon, oil, vinegar and spices and pour over mixture, stirring well. Serve as it is or refrigerate and serve cold. This salad makes a great stuffing for tomatoes, green or red peppers, stuffed in pita bread, or rolled in whole-wheat flour tortillas.

Greek Salad

Another hit in my cooking classes! This is a delicious beautiful salad that's flavored well. Use the special dressing or a vinaigrette.

> 1 bunch red leaf or green leaf lettuce, torn in small pieces
> 1 small cucumber, cut in chunks
> 1 red pepper, cut in chunks
> ¹/₂ cup black olives, cut lengthwise (optional)
> 1 small white onion, chopped fine
> 2 small Roma tomatoes, chopped

Wash and peel cucumber and chop vegetables. Toss ingredients together and serve with dressing.

Dressing:

> 2 tablespoons olive oil
> 2 tablespoons lemon juice
> 2 cloves garlic, minced
> 1 teaspoon each: sea salt, parsley, paprika
> ¹/₂ teaspoon basil
> 2 teaspoons oregano
> dash cayenne

Mix ingredients and blend.

Grilled Chicken Caesar Salad

Eating a salad with some protein makes a perfect start for a meal. Serve with a slice of whole-grain bread.

Dressing:

> 1 clove garlic
> 3 tablespoons Spectrum olive oil
> 2 tablespoons lemon juice
> 1 teaspoon Dijon mustard
> dash sea salt or salt substitute

Salad:
1 head Romaine lettuce
6-8 strips of grilled chicken
1 cup garlic croutons (see recipe below)
Parmesan cheese

Mince fine, press, or crush garlic. Add oil, lemon juice, mustard and salt and mix together.

Wash and dry lettuce and break into bite-size pieces. Add to bowl and toss. Top with Parmesan cheese and garlic croutons.

Crouton recipe: 1 slice whole-wheat toast, 1 tablespoon Spectrum olive oil or Pam cooking spray, 1 clove garlic, and whole-wheat bread slices. Rub both sides of toast with clove of garlic and gently brush oil or spray with cooking spray. Keep warm. Cube and toss in salad.

Most meat markets or grocery stores carry prepared grilled chicken strips.

Healthy Coleslaw (Mary June Parks)

Mary June's coleslaw is a healthy version of a basic coleslaw recipe.

1 cup each: red and white cabbage, shredded
1 medium carrot, grated
2 tablespoons apple cider vinegar
3 tablespoons olive oil
1 tablespoon honey

Blend liquids and sprinkle over slaw. Serve chilled.
(Used with permission.)

Mexican Taco (Tempeh) Salad

Another healthy version of a favorite salad. There are two spice combinations available: Hain Taco Seasoning Mix and Santa Fe Taco Mix. Both can be used with either beef, chicken, turkey or tempeh. If you want to make your own seasoning mix, combine equal parts of chili, garlic, basil, cumin, oregano, ginger, parsley and cayenne. Using tempeh makes it a low-fat salad.

8 ounces tempeh, grated (or equal parts of beef, chicken, or turkey strips)
$^1/_2$ medium onion
1 package Taco seasoning mix
1 head Green leaf lettuce
$^1/_2$ cabbage, shredded
1 16-ounce can kidney beans, drained
3 carrots, chopped
1 tomato, chopped
$^1/_3$ cup Tofu Rella cheddar cheese, grated (find at health food store)

Grate tempeh with a cheese grater. Saute tempeh in a saucepan sprayed with vegetable spray. Add onion, Taco seasoning mix, and water. Mix and cook, stirring 5-10 minutes. Meanwhile, combine cabbage, kidney beans, carrots, tomatoes and cheese. Top with Taco seasoning mixture.

If you want a dressing, here's a nice one:

Vinegar dressing: 2 tablespoons olive oil, $^1/_3$ cup brown rice vinegar, 1 teaspoon chili powder, and 1 teaspoon cumin. Blend well and pour over salad.

Oriental Salad

Here's a nice way to have a crunchy, tasty salad for variety.

10 stalks asparagus, canned or steamed 10 minutes
14 snow peas
1 stalk celery, slice on angle
$^1/_2$ can bamboo shoots, rinsed and dried
$^1/_2$ can water chestnuts, drained
$^1/_4$ cup onion, chopped

Mix ingredients and serve with favorite dressing.

Romaine and Asparagus Salad

The green romaine, asparagus and parsley make this salad a wonderful source of calcium. Nice and crunchy, too.

> 1 head Romaine lettuce
> 4 stalks asparagus
> $1/2$ cup red cabbage, shredded fine
> 2 stalks celery
> $1/2$ bunch parsley

Clean, chop and toss with basic vinegar dressing or: $1/4$ cup olive oil, juice of 1 lemon, 1 clove garlic, minced and 1 teaspoon thyme.

BEAN, RICE AND VEGETABLE DISHES

Baked Kidney Beans

Simple, easy and delicious!

> 1 cup kidney beans
> 4 cups water
> 2 onions, quartered
> 1 clove garlic
> dash sea salt, cayenne

Wash kidney beans well and soak overnight in 4 cups water. Bring to a boil, skim off foam. Add onions and garlic and place in a 350°F. oven for 1-2 hours or until beans are soft. Add seasoning to taste.

Basic Brown Rice

An easy recipe for perfect rice. Don't lift the lid while cooking.

> 1 cup brown rice
> 2 cups water
> salt to season ($1/4$ to $1/2$ teaspoon)

Wash, rinse and drain rice. Put rice in a saucepan and add water. Bring water to a boil, low heat and simmer 55 minutes. Add to soups, casseroles, salads, or add stir fried vegetables.

Greek Lentils

This is one of my students' favorite dishes in my cooking classes. Lentils are one of the easiest beans to digest and these herbs and spices make a great dish or side dish.

> 1 cup dried lentils
> 2 tablespoons Dijon mustard
> $^{1}/_{4}$ teaspoon oregano
> $^{1}/_{2}$ teaspoon cumin
> 2 tablespoons olive oil
> 1 onion, minced
> 1 teaspoon sea salt
> **Optional:** ripe olives, Feta cheese

Wash and rinse lentils. Add 2 cups of water and bring to a boil. Cover and simmer for 30 minutes. Let cool and drain off water. In a separate bowl, combine spices and stir well. Pour over lentils and mix well. These lentils can be served hot or cold. Other ideas: Add cooked pasta to make a pasta-lentil salad. Make a Greek taco by using this mixture on a corn or flour tortilla.

Oatmeal

Oatmeal is a wonderful grain for breakfast, since it's a complex carbohydrate it will stick to your ribs and hold you over until lunch.

> $^{2}/_{3}$ cups rolled oats
> $1^{1}/_{2}$ cups water
> $^{1}/_{2}$ cup raisins
> $^{1}/_{2}$ teaspoon cinnamon

Bring water to a boil, add oats and raisins, cinnamon, salt and reduce heat to low, simmering 5-10 minutes or until thick. Serve hot with soy milk, rice milk, honey or maple syrup.

Variations: substitute $^{1}/_{2}$ cup dates for raisins

Oriental Wild Rice

This is great! Brown rice and wild rice team up for a wonderfully flavored rice/vegetable dish. Serve with a salad and whole grain bread.

1 cup cooked brown rice
½ cup wild rice
3 cups water or vegetable stock
1 teaspoon sea salt
½ cup mushrooms, sliced
2 stalks celery, chopped
1 onion, chopped
Vegetable spray
dash cayenne
1 teaspoon soy sauce

Saute onion, celery and mushrooms in a saucepan sprayed with vegetable spray a few minutes. Add liquid, wild rice and sea salt and bring to a boil. Lower heat and simmer for 20 minutes. Add cooked brown rice and heat.

Simple Bean Chili

Quick, low fat and delicious!

1 cup pinto beans, cooked
2 cloves garlic, minced
1 can tomatoes, crushed
2 tablespoons chili powder

Add spices and tomatoes to cooked beans and simmer covered for 30 minutes. Serve with a small side salad and corn bread.

Spicy Black Beans

A delicious bean dish.

$^1/_2$ teaspoon olive oil
1 small onion, minced
1 clove garlic, minced
4 carrots, chopped
2 cans black beans drained (or cooked from scratch)
1 cup corn, drained
1 teaspoon sea salt
$^1/_2$ teaspoon cumin
$^1/_4$ teaspoon white pepper

Saute onion and garlic in oil or vegetable spray. Add carrots and saute until tender. Add black beans, corn, and seasonings. Cook until heated through, about 5 minutes. Serve with brown rice and salad.

Vegetable Chop Suey

My students in the cooking classes loved this simple, delicious and healthy dish. You can make it a meal by adding chicken.

Sauce:

$^3/_4$ cup vegetable broth
1 tablespoon Tamari soy sauce (low sodium)
1 teaspoon honey
1 teaspoon brown rice vinegar
1 tablespoon arrowroot or corn starch diluted in 3 tablespoons water
1 small onion, sliced in crescent shapes
$^1/_2$ cup celery, sliced diagonally
$^1/_2$ cup green cabbage, sliced or grated
1 cup mushrooms, sliced
1 green pepper, sliced diagonally
2 carrots, sliced diagonally
$^1/_2$ cup water chestnuts

Combine ingredients for sauce in a bowl and put aside. Meanwhile, chop vegetables and lightly sauté in a saucepan sprayed with vegetable spray, or "water saute" by adding $1/4$ cup water and stirring over low heat. Start with onions and add celery, cabbage, carrots, mushrooms, green peppers and water chestnuts. When vegetables are still slightly crisp, add sauce mixture and simmer 10-15 minutes until slightly thick. Serve over cooked brown rice, cooked brown rice noodles, or cooked Oriental noodles. For cooking noodles, follow recipe on package.

FISH AND CHICKEN DISHES

Chicken Cacciatore

A quick, tasty, fairly low-fat recipe.

> 4 boneless chicken breasts
> 2 cups tomato puree (no sugar, low salt)
> 1 cup green pepper, chopped
> 1 cup mushrooms, chopped
> 1 cup onions, chopped
> 1 tablespoon Canola oil or Pam cooking spray
> $1/4$ teaspoon white pepper
> 1 clove garlic
> 1 teaspoon oregano and paprika

Sauté chicken breasts in Pam or oil until brown. Put aside. Sauté onion, mushrooms, green peppers and spices. Add tomato puree and bring to a boil and stir until thick. Add chicken and simmer together 5 minutes. Spoon sauce over chicken when you serve it.

Chicken Italian Style

A delicious meal in one pan. Serve with a slice of whole grain bread.

> 2 whole chicken breasts, boned and skinned
> 1 tablespoon olive oil
> $1/2$ lb. sliced mushrooms
> 1 medium onion, chopped
> 2 red or green peppers, chopped

2 cloves garlic, chopped
4-5 tomatoes, chopped
$1/4$ teaspoon each: parsley, oregano, thyme, marjoram

Brown chicken in oil; add garlic and onions and sauté until tender. Add mushrooms, peppers, and tomatoes and cook on low for 3 minutes. You can add corn starch or arrowroot powder dissolved in $1/2$ cup water to thicken. Let mixture simmer for 20 minutes. You can add sea salt or soy sauce for flavor.

Chicken Oriental Stir-fry

If you're tired of grilled chicken, here's a nice variation.

2 large chicken breasts, cut in strips
$1/2$ head Chinese cabbage or Savoy cabbage
4 stalks celery, slice on slant
4 green onions, chopped in slant
1 stalk broccoli, chopped
1 cup pea pods
sliced water chestnuts
1-2 carrots, sliced diagonally
2 cloves garlic, minced
$1/4$ cup water
$1/4$ cup Tamari soy sauce
3 teaspoons corn starch or arrowroot powder

Slowly heat 1 tablespoon canola oil in a wok and brown chicken strips. Sauté garlic and onions. Add all the vegetables except for sprouts and cook quickly until tender, over lower heat. Add remaining vegetables and continue to cook. Separately mix together corn starch or arrowroot powder and $1/4$ cup water. Then add to vegetables and stir over low heat. Add soy sauce and serve.

Herbed Chicken

> $^1/_2$ lb. boneless chicken
> 2 tablespoons frozen orange juice concentrate
> 1 teaspoon oregano
> $^1/_4$ teaspoon parsley
> 1 teaspoon basil
> $^1/_2$ teaspoon lemon juice
> $^1/_4$ teaspoon mustard

Preheat broiler and broil chicken. Mix ingredients in a bowl and brush half the mixture over chicken. Broil 10 minutes or until chicken is browned. Base with remaining mixture. Broil 10 minutes longer.

Optional: 1 tablespoon lemon juice, $^1/_2$ teaspoon garlic, 1 teaspoon Dijon.

Dijon Perch

A wonderful flavorful way to prepare perch.

> 4 perch fillets
> $^1/_4$ cup Dijon mustard
> 2 tablespoons lemon juice
> 2 tablespoons water
> 1 teaspoon white pepper
> 1 teaspoon thyme
> 2 tomatoes, chopped

Rinse fish with cold water and pat dry with a paper towel. Place fish on a baking sheet and sprinkle with white pepper. Combine mustard, water, thyme, and tomatoes well and pour over fish. Seal with aluminum foil. Bake at 450°F. for 15-20 minutes or until fish flakes easily when tested. Remove from foil and serve.

Easy Baked or Grilled Fish

An easy way to prepare most light fish.

> 4 4-oz. cod or whitefish fillets
> 2 tablespoons Spectrum olive oil
> dash Hain sea salt
> dash cayenne pepper
> 1 tablespoon minced parsley
> 1/4 cup green onion, minced
> 2 cloves garlic, minced
> 2 tablespoon lemon juice

Preheat oven to 400°F. Spray baking pan with Pam cooking spray or brush with olive oil and place fish. Mix remaining ingredients in a bowl and pour over fish mixture. Bake for 15-20 minutes until fish is flaky.

Easy Salmon Bake

An easy way to use canned or fresh fish.

> 1 4-oz. can Salmon (or tuna)
> 2 tablespoons olive oil
> sea salt
> dash cayenne pepper
> 1/4 cup green onion, minced
> 2 cloves garlic, minced
> 2 tablespoons lemon juice

Mix everything together and put into a baking dish. Bake at 350°F. for 15 minutes.

Lemon Baked Halibut

You can use this recipe for any light fish. Serve with steamed vegetables or a salad.

> 5 halibut fillets
> 1 tablespoon finely minced garlic
> 1 tablespoon lemon juice
> $1/2$ teaspoon sea salt

Sprinkle garlic, lemon juice, and salt over halibut and bake in a covered pan in a 350°F. oven for 20 minutes.

Additional Resources

BROCHURES

"Snack Your Way to Five a Day" To receive other brochures that can help you reach the goal of five or more servings of fruits and vegetables every day, or for more information on diet and cancer, call the Cancer Information Service: 1-800-4-CANCER.

GOVERNMENT PUBLICATIONS

"The Food Guide Pyramid," U.S.D.A. Human Nutrition Information Service, August 1992, Leaflet No. 572.

To order a copy of "The Food Guide Pyramid" booklet, send a $1.00 check or money order made out to the Superintendent of Documents to: Consumer Information Center, Department 159-Y, Pueblo, Colorado 81009.

"How To Read The New Food Label," Food and Drug Administration, FDA 93-2260.

"Good Sources of Nutrients," USDA, January 1990.

"Dietary Guidelines for Americans," U.S. Department of Agriculture, U.S. Department of Health and Human Services, Fourth Edition, 1995.

NEWSLETTERS/MAGAZINES

Nutrition Action Healthletter
Center for Science in the Public Interest
Suite 300, 1875 Connecticut Avenue N.W.
Washington, DC 20009-5728

Health Alert
Dr. Bruce West
5 Harris Court, N6
Monterey, CA 93940-5753

Natural Health Magazine
P.O. Box 7440
Red Oak, IA 51591-4440

Total Health Magazine
165 North 100 East, Suite 2
St. George, UT 84770-9964

Vegetarian Times
P.O. Box 446
Mount Morris, IL 61054
800-435-9610

FOOD SOURCES

Stevia Products
Stevia can be purchased at your local health food store or through the following companies:
Stevita
Arlington, TX
1-817-483-0044

Body Ecology
1-800-511-2660

Now Natural Foods
Chicago, IL
1-800-999-8069

Allergies
The Food Allergy Network
1-703-691-3179

Organically Grown Coffee
Cafe Altura
Clean Food, Inc.
760 East Santa Maria St.
Santa Papula, CA 93060
1-800-526-8328

Coffee Substitutes

Pero Instant Natural Beverage
P. O. Box 25846
Salt Lake City, UT 84125-0846

Postum Instant Hot Beverage
Maxwell House Coffee Company
Kraft General Foods, Inc.
Box PR7
White Plains, NY 10625
1-800-432-6333

Teecino Caffe, Inc.
P. O. Box 42259
Santa Barbara, CA 93105
1-800-498-3434

Herbal Tea Companies

Celestial Seasonings
4600 Sleepytime Dr.
Boulder, CO 80301-3292
1-800-351-8175

The Republic of Tea
8 Digital Drive, Suite 100
Novato, CA 94949-5759
1-800-298-TEA

Hormone Saliva Test Kit

Aeron Labs
San Leandro, CA
1-800-631-7900

Soy Foods

The United Soybean Board
1-800-825-5769

Mori-Nu Tofu
1-800-445-3350

HEALTH PROFESSIONALS

Chiropractic
American Chiropractic Association
1701 Clarendon Boulevard
Arlington, VA 22209
(703) 276-8800
(800) 986-4636
www.americhiro.org

International Chiropractor Association
1110 N. Glebe Road, Suite 1000
Arlington, VA 22201
(800) 423-4690
www.chiropractic.org
Email: chiro@chiropractic.org

Osteopathic
American Osteopathic Association
142 East Ontario Street
Chicago, IL 60611
(312) 202-8000
www.AOA-net.org

Naturopathic
American Association of Naturopathic Physicians
601 Valley, Suite 105
Seattle, Washington 98109
(206) 298-0126
www.naturopathic.org

Naturopathic medical schools are accredited by the Council on Naturopathic Medical Education which is recognized by the United States Department of Education as the specialty accreditation body for this field.

There are two levels of CNME accreditation: fully accredited institution and candidate for accreditation. National College of Naturopathic Medicine and Bastyr University are fully accredited. Southwest College of Naturopathic Medicine and Canadian College of Naturopathic Medicine are candidates for accreditation.

National College of Naturopathic Medicine
049 Southwest Porter Avenue
Portland, OR 97201
(503) 499-4343
www.ncnm.edu

Bastyr University
14500 Juanita Drive
Kenmore, WA 98028
(425) 823-1300
www.bastyr.edu

Southwest College of Naturopathic Medicine
2140 E. Broadway Road
Tempe, AZ 85282
(480) 858-9100
www.scnn.edu

Canadian College of Naturopathic Medicine
1255 Shepherd Avenue East
North York, Ontario
Canada M2K 1E2
(416) 498-1255

Medical Doctors

American College for Advancement in Medicine (ACAM)
23121 Verdugo Drive, Suite 204
Laguna Hills, CA 92653
www.acam.org

American Holistic Health Association (AHHA)
P. O. Box 17400
Anaheim, CA 92817
(714) 779-6152
ahha.org

Nutritional Dentistry

Donald W. Warren, D.D.S.
Rt 6, Box 152
Clinton, AR 72031
(501) 745-4656
(501) 745-6317

Dr. Warren has a dental practice that integrates designed clinical nutrition.

NUTRITION INFORMATION

Training as a Certified Nutritionist, which is a two-year program, requires that you first have an undergraduate degree. Three-hour exams follow all course work, and continuing education requirements are expected yearly to keep the C.N. license. There are several type of nutritionist training programs, most of which require at least an undergraduate degree, and often a Master's Degree with requirements for continuing education. I have been impressed with the quality of the C.N.s, C.C.N.s and C.N.S.s I have met at NNFA meetings around the country. But before you begin working with any nutritionist, or N.D., get several references and ask if they are certified.

American Health Sciences University AHSU
1010 S. Joliet, Suite 107
Aurora, CO 80012
(800) 530-8079
www.ahsu.com

Society of Certified Nutritionists (SCN)
2111 Bridgeport Way W. #2
University Place, WA 98466
(800) 342-8037
www.certifiednutritionist.com
International and American Association of Clinical Nutritionists
(IAACN)
1677 Addison Road
Dallas, TX 75248
972-407-9089

Association of California Nutritional Consultants (ACNC)
39149 Guardino Drive
Fremont, CA 94538
510-693-7823

Life Design Nutrition
Lorrie Medford, C.N.
P.O. Box 54007
Tulsa, OK 74155
Lorrie@lifedesignnutrition.com
918-664-4483
www.lifedesignnutrition.com

Note: I have several friends who are Registered Dieticians and I appreciate their education and the work they are doing to educate the public. However, most dietitians don't recommend the use of nutritional food supplements, believing that we can get most of our nutrition from foods. You can easily find an R.D. by phoning your local hospital. If you are looking for specific information on nutritional supplements, ask them about their knowledge of supplements when you call them.

FOOD INFORMATION

American Soybean Association
540 Maryville Centre Drive, #390
St. Louise, MO 63141-9200
800-TALK SOY (800-825-5769)
www.soyfoods.com

Health Food Stores

Whenever I am in Dallas, Houston, or a number of larger cities, I try to stop at one of these markets. Perhaps there is a one near you. If you do not have a local health food store in your area, you can order from these markets on the Internet.

Whole Foods Market
Whole Foods is one of the largest natural foods chains that carries

organic produce, baked goods, a deli and supermarket.
www.wholefoods.com

Wild Oats
Another large natural foods chain that carries a complete line of herbs
and supplements. You will be delighted with their large selection of
organic foods, skin care products, and full-service deli.
www.wildoats.com

Endnotes

Chapter One

1. Bob Schwartz, *Diets Still Don't Work* (Houston, TX: Breakthru Publishing, 1990), p. 3.

Chapter Two

1. Lindsey Duncan, C.N., N.D. "Internal Detoxification" *Healthy & Natural Journal,* October 1988.

Chapter Three

1. Jonn Matsen, N.D., *The Mysterious Cause of Illness* (Canfield, OH: Fischer Publishing, 1987), pp. 7-9.
2. Cass Ingram, D.O., *Self-Test Nutrition Guide* (Buffalo Grove, IL: Knowledge House Publishers, 1994), p. 162.
3. Ingram, p. 162.
4. Ingram, p. 163.
5. Ibid.
6. *Tulsa World*, Aug. 29, 1995, p. 12.

Chapter Four

1. Bernard Jensen, D.C., Ph.D., *Tissue Cleansing Through Bowel Management* (Escondido, CA: Bernard Jensen, 1981), p. 3.
2. Lindsey Duncan, C.N., N.D. "Internal Detoxification" *Healthy & Natural Journal,* October 1988.
3. Amy Steeves interview, May 17, 1998.
4. Robert Gray, *The Colon Health Handbook* (Reno, NV: Emerald Publishing, 1980), p. 25.
5. Amy Steeves interview, May 17, 1998.

Chapter Five

1. Jonn Matsen, N.D., *The Mysterious Cause of Illness* (Canfield, OH: Fischer Publishing, 1987), p. 42.
2. Matsen, p. 51.
3. Jonathan V. Wright, M.D., *Dr. Wright's Guide to Healing With Nutrition* (New Canaan, CT: Keats Publishing, Inc., 1984), pp. 51-52.
4. Matsen, pp. 45-46.
5. Willa Vae Bowles, "How To Purify Your Bloodstream," *Total Health* Magazine, (February 1987), p. 34.
6. Marilyn and Harvey Diamond, *Fit for Life* (New York, NY: Warner Books, 1985), p. 67.
7. John A. McDougall, M.D., *The McDougall Plan* (Hampton, NJ: New Win Publishing, Inc., 1985), p. 18.
8. Willa Vae Bowles, "Be Good To Your Liver," *Total Health* Magazine, (June 1992), pp. 30-32.

Chapter Six

1. Louise Tenney, *Modern Day Plagues,* Revised (Pleasant Grove, UT: Woodland Books, 1994) p. 320.
2. Cass Ingram, D.O., *Self Test-Nutrition Guide* (Buffalo Grove, IL: Knowledge House Publishers, 1994), p. 250.
3. Dr. James Balch and Phyllis, *Prescription for Nutritional Healing* (Garden City Park, NY: Avery Publishing, 1990), p. 213.
4. Ingram, Cass, D.O., *How to Eat Right and Live Longer* (Buffalo Grove, IL: Knowledge House Publishers, 1989), p. 79.
5. Brian Scott Peskin, *Beyond the Zone* (Houston, TX: Noble Publishing, 1999), p. 218.
6. "Complete Junk," *Nutrition Action Healthletter*, Vol. 25, No. 4 (May 1988), p. 16.

Chapter Seven

1. Nancy Appleton, Ph.D., *Lick the Sugar Habit* (Garden City Park, NY: Avery Publishing Group, 1988), p. 21.
2. Cass Ingram, D.O., *How to Eat Right and Live Longer* (Buffalo Grove, IL: Knowledge House Publishers, 1989), p. 119.
3. Appleton, pp. 24-25.
4. Jonn Matsen, D.O., *The Mysterious Cause of Illness* (Canfield, OH: Fischer Publishing, 1987), p. 113.

5. Dr. James Balch and Phyllis, *Prescription for Nutritional Healing* (Garden City Park, NY: Avery Publishing, 1990), p. 79.

Chapter Eight

1. H. Leighton Steward, Dr. Morrison C. Bethea, Dr. Samuel S. Andrews and Dr. Luis A. Balart, *Sugar Busters!* (New York, NY: The Ballantine Publishing Group, 1998), p. 18.
2. Mark Messina, Ph.D. and Virginia Messina, R.D., *The Simple Soybean and Your Health,* (Garden City Park, NY: Avery Publishing, 1994), p. 111.
3. Dr. Bruce West, *Disease and Prevention,* (Monterey, CA, 1995), p. 14.

Chapter Nine

1. Dr. William G. Crook, *The Yeast Connection: A Medical Breakthrough* (Jackson, TN: Professional Books, 1983), pp. 15, 30-33.
2. Lindsey Duncan, C.N., N.D., "Candida Self-Test." *Healthy & Natural Journal*, JS 10073-00.

Chapter Ten

1. Hulda Regehr Clark, Ph.D., N.D., *The Cure For All Diseases* (San Diego, CA: ProMotion Publishing, 1995), p. 377.

Chapter Eleven

1. John R. Lee, M.D., *What Your Doctor May Not Tell You About Menopause* (New York: Warner Books, 1996), p. 34.
2. Lee, p. 71.
3. Cynthia Drasler, phone interview, April 1998.
4. Raquel Martin, *The Estrogen Alternative* (Rochester, VT: Healing Arts Press, 1997), p. 12.
5. Cynthia Drasler, phone interview, April 1998.
6. Raquel Martin, p. 47.

Chapter Twelve

1. Lisa Messinger, *Why Should I Eat Better?* (Garden City Park, NY: Avery Publishers), 1993, p. 1.
2. Myles T. Bader, Dr., *4001 Food Facts and Chef's Secrets* (San Diego, CA: Mylin Enterprises, 1992), p. 241.

3. Mary June Parks, *A New You* (Frankfort, KY: Parks Publishers, 1982), p. 24.

4. *Talking Food* pamphlet entitled: "Sugar and How it Gets That Way," Charlestown, MA, 1977.

5. Nancy Appleton, Ph.D., *Lick the Sugar Habit* (Garden City Park, NY: Avery Publishers, 1988), pp. 78-96.

6. Mary June Parks, *Menu and the Mind* (Frankfort, KY: Parks Publishers, 1986), pp. 65-68.

7. Parks, pp. 65, 71.

8. Appleton, p. 9.

9. Robert Crayhon, M.S., *Nutrition Made Simple* (New York: M. Evans & Company, Inc., 1994) p. 57.

10. Brian Scott Peskin, *Beyond the Zone* (Houston, TX: Noble Publishing, 1999), p. 182.

11. Steven C. Strauss and Gail North, *The Body Signal Secret* (Emmaus, PA: Rodale Press, 1991), p. 181.

12. Andrew Weil, M.D., *8 Weeks to Optimum Health* (New York: Alfred A. Knopf, 1997), p. 238.

Chapter Fourteen

1. Udo Erasmus, *Fats That Heal/Fats That Kill* (Burnaby, BC: Alive Books, 1993), p. 343.

2. Brian Scott Peskin, *Beyond the Zone* (Houston, TX: Noble Publishing, 1999), p. 11.

3. Peskin, p. 21.

4. *Talking Food* pamphlet: "Vegetable Oil: The Unsaturated Facts" Charlestown, MA, 1977.

5. Peskin, p. 72.

6. Peskin, p. 121.

7. Peskin, p. 45.

8. Peskin, p. 127.

9. Peskin, p. 197.

10. Peskin, p. 67.

11. "Trans: The Phantom Fat," *Nutrition Action Healthletter*, Vol. 23, No. 7 (September, 1996), pp. 10-11.

12. Robert Crayhon, M.S., *Nutrition Made Simple* (New York: M. Evans & Company, Inc., 1994), p. 52.

Chapter Fifteen

1. "The Dietary Goals for the United States: Select Committee on Nutrition and Human Needs," (February 1977), U. S. Government Printing Office, Washington D.C., p. 13.
2. Bill Pearl, *Getting Stronger* (Bolimas, CA: Shelter Publishing), pp. 398-399.
3. T. Colin Campbell, Ph.D., *The China Project: Inside Our Living Laboratory* (Ithaca, NY: New Century Nutrition, 1996), p. 23.
4. Campbell, p. 5.
5. Campbell, p. 10-25.
6. Campbell, p. 18.
7. Brian Scott Peskin, *Beyond the Zone* (Houston, TX: Noble Publishing, 1999), p. 237.
8. Campbell, p. 10.
9. Campbell, pp. 17-18.
10. John McDougall, M.D., *The McDougall Plan* (Hampton, NJ: New Win Publishing, Inc., 1985), p. 49-55.
11. Ellen Buchman Ewald, *Recipes for a Small Planet* (New York, NY: Ballantine Books, 1973), pp. 12-15.

Chapter Sixteen

1. Stephen Cherniske, M.S., *Caffeine Blues* (New York: NY, Warner Books, 1998), p. 36, 39.
2. Cherniske, pp. 285-293.

Chapter Eighteen

1. Peter D'Adamo, M.D., *Eat Right for Your Type* (New York, NY: G. P. Putnam and Sons, 1997).
2. Patrick Quillin, Ph.D., *Beating Cancer With Nutrition* (Tulsa, OK: The Nutrition Times Press, Inc., 1994), p. 85.
3. Quillin, p. 85.
4. Ibid.

Chapter Twenty-One

1. Dr. Bruce West, "Health Facts for the New Millennium," (Carmel, CA: *Health Alert,* 1996), p. 5.

Appendix B: Benefits of Apple Cider Vinegar

1. Paul C. Bragg, *Apple Cider Vinegar: Miracle Health System* (Santa Barbara, CA: Health Science forty-sixth printing), p. 7.

Glossary

Acidophilus: (Lactobacillus): A type of "friendly" bacteria that lives in our intestines. They help promote proper elimination, aid in energy production, reduce blood cholesterol levels, and assist in correcting yeast overgrowth. Found in yogurt and kefir cultures.

Adrenals: Two small glands located on top of the kidneys. An energy-producing gland, the adrenals help regulate sugar and carbohydrate metabolism, are involved in sex hormone production, and help the body to handle stress.

Amylase: Enzymes secreted by the pancreas and salivary glands that break down carbohydrates.

Antioxidant: Substances that neutralize free radicals.

Arachidonic acid: A polyunsaturated fatty acid, which is a precursor of prostaglandins essential in nutrition.

Candida Albicans: A yeast organism that normally lives in the mouth and intestinal tract. A series of problems occur when this yeast over-grows in the intestines: poor digestion, fatigue, bloating, gas, poor elimination, and carbohydrate cravings.

Carcinogen: A substance that can cause cancer.

Cholecystokinin: A hormone secreted by the mucosa of the upper intestinal tract which stimulates contraction of the gallbladder.

Colonics: A method of irrigating the colon to help cleanse the colon wall of impacted material.

Digestive Enzymes: An enzyme that promotes the breakdown of proteins, fats and carbohydrates in the digestive system.

Edema: Excessive fluid retention.

Ephedra (ephedrine): A stimulant of the central nervous system, often used in weight-loss formulas to increase metabolism. Caution should be used by anyone with thyroid problems, diabetes, adrenal insufficiency, or high blood pressure.

Essential Oils (Essential Fatty Acids): Essential oils that are not produced by the body and are required for healthy hair, skin, mucous membranes, nerves, thyroid, adrenals, and development of hormones.

Estrogen: A female hormone produced by the ovaries responsible for female sexual characteristics.

Fibroids: Fleshy growths in the uterus or breast.

Gastro-intestinal: Pertaining to the stomach and intestines.

Genistein: A phytochemical found in soy foods, which has been proven anti-cancerous.

Glucagon: A hormone secreted by the pancreas that helps regulate blood sugar and helps promote fat burning.

Glycemic Index: A rating of foods according to how quickly they are converted to glucose, the form of sugar in the blood.

Goitrogens: Foods which can induce an iodine deficiency often found in the cruciferous family: cabbage, rutabaga, and broccoli.

Hydrochloric Acid (HCl): A colorless, compound of hydrogen chloride (HCl); the acid secreted by the stomach to facilitate digestion.

Hydrogenation: The addition of hydrogen molecules to unsaturated oils which is proven detrimental to cells.

Hypoglycemia: A low-blood sugar level.

Hypothyroid: Underactive thyroid, generally from an iodine deficiency. Symptoms include weight gain, depression, fatigue and cold hands and feet.

Insulin: A hormone secreted by the pancreas that lowers blood glucose by directing cells to use glucose.

Lactose: A sugar in cow's milk.

Lipase: The enzyme that breaks down fat; secreted by the pancreas.

Menopause: The time period when a women's cycle ends.

Miso: A soy product; soybean paste made from soybeans that have been fermented for 18 months to 3 years; used medicinally and as a flavoring in Japanese cooking. High in salt; not for sodium-restricted diets.

Osteoporosis: Refers to the loss of bone mineral density.

Probiotics: The bacteria found in healthy bacteria, the primary health-promoting bacteria is lactobacilli and bifido bacteria.

Progesterone: A female hormone produced by the ovaries which has proven benefits for bone-density health.

Protease: The enzyme that breaks down protein.

Psyllium: An effective intestinal cleanser and stool softener found in many colon cleanse products.

Serotonin: A neurotransmitter made from tryptophan.

Tempeh: A soybean mixture; made from pressing soybeans and rice and allowing this mixture to ferment. Sold in cakes, it can be grated or grilled for an entree. Very high in protein and low in saturated fat.

Thermogenics: The name for substances that stimulate the body's ability to burn excess calories which would be stored as fat.

Tofu: A type of cheese made from soy milk.

Tryptophan: An amino acid that aids in the conversion of serotonin, found in protein foods like turkey, chicken, seeds and nuts.

Bibliography

Appleton, Nancy. Ph.D. *Lick the Sugar Habit.* (Garden City Park, NY: Avery Publishing Group,1988).

Bader, Myles T. Dr. *4001 Food Facts and Chef's Secrets.* (San Diego, CA: Mylin Enterprises, 1992).

Balch, James, M.D. and Phyllis. *Prescription for Nutritional Healing.* (Garden City Park, NY: Avery Publishing, 1990).

Bateson-Koch, Carolee, D.C. *Allergies Disease in Disguise.* (Burnaby, B.C. Canada: Alive Books, 1994).

Block, Mary Ann, M.D. *No More Ritalin: Treating ADHD Without Drugs.* (New York, NY: Kensington Books, 1996).

Bragg, Paul C. *Apple Cider Vinegar: Miracle Health System.* (Santa Barbara, CA: Health Science, forty-sixth printing).

Calbom, Cheri and Keane, Maureen. *Juicing for Life.* (Garden City Park, NY: Avery Publishing Group, 1992).

Campbell, T. Colin, Ph.D. and Cox, Christine. *The China Project: Inside Our Living Laboratory.* (Ithaca, NY: New Century Nutrition, 1996).

Challem, Jack and Dolby, Victoria. *Homocysteine: The New "Cholesterol."* (New Canaan, CT: Keats Publishing, Inc., 1996).

Cherniske, Stephen, M.S. *Caffeine Blues.* (New York: NY: Warner Books, 1998).

Cichoke, Anthony J., D.C. *Enzymes and Enzyme Therapy.* (New Canaan, CT: Keats Publishing, Inc., 1994).

Cichoke, Anthony J., D.C. *The Complete Book of Enzyme Therapy.* (Garden City Park, NY: Avery Publishing Group, 1999).

Clark, Hulda Regehr, Ph.D., N.D. *The Cure for All Diseases.* (San Diego, CA: ProMotion Publishing, 1995).

Crayhon, Robert, M.S. *Nutrition Made Simple.* (New York, NY: M. Evans and Company, Inc., 1994).

Crook, William G., M.D. *The Yeast Connection: A Medical Breakthrough.* (Jackson, TN: Professional Books, 1983).

Crook, William G., M.D. *Tracking Down Hidden Food Allergies.* (Jackson, TN: Professional Books, 1980. Eighth printing, 1991).

D'Adamo, Peter, M.D. *Eat Right for Your Type.* (New York, NY: G.P. Putnam and Sons, 1997).

DesMaisons, Kathleen, Ph.D. *Potatoes Not Prozac.* (New York, NY: Simon & Schuster, 1998).

Diamond, Harvey and Marilyn. *Fit for Life.* (New York, NY: Warner Books, 1985).

Dufty, William. *Sugar Blues.* (New York, NY: Warner Books, 1975).

Elrod, Joe M. Dr. *Reversing Fibromyalgia.* Pleasant Grove, UT: Woodland Publishing, 1997).

Erasmus, Udo. *Fats That Heal/Fats That Kill.* (Burnaby, B.C.: Alive Books, 1993).

Ewald, Ellen Buchman. *Recipes for a Small Planet.* (New York, NY: Ballantine Books, 1973).

Gates, Donna. *The Body Ecology Diet.* (Atlanta, GA: B.E.D. Publications, 1993).

Gates, Donna. *The Stevia Story.* (Atlanta, GA: B.E.D. Publications, 1997).

Gioannini, Marilyn. *Food Allergy Cookbook.* (Rocklin, CA: Prima Publishing, 1996.)

Gittleman, Ann Louise, M.S. *Get the Sugar Out.* (Garden City Park, NY: Avery Publishing, 1993).

Gittleman, Ann Louise, M.S. *Super Nutrition for Menopause. (*Garden City Park, NY: Avery Publishing Group, 1998).

Gray, Robert. *The Colon Health Handbook.* (Reno, NV: Emerald Publishing, 1980. Twelfth Revised Edition).

Hagler, Louise. *Tofu Quick and Easy.* (Summertown, TN: Book Publishing Co., 1986).

Howell, Edward. *Enzyme Nutrition.* (Garden City Park, NY: Avery Publishers Group, 1985).

Hurt Jones, Marjorie, R.N. *The Allergy Self-Help Cookbook.* (Emmaus, PA: Rodale Press, 1984).

Ingram, Cass, D.O. *Self-Test Nutrition Guide.* (Buffalo Grove, IL: Knowledge House Publishers, 1994).

Ingram, Cass, D.O. *How to Eat Right and Live Longer.* (Buffalo Grove, IL: Knowledge House Publishers, 1989).

Jensen, Bernard D.C., Ph.D. *Tissue Cleansing Through Bowel Management.* (Escondido, CA: Bernard Jensen, 1981).

Lee, John R., M.D. *What Your Doctor May Not Tell You About Menopause.* (New York, NY: Warner Books, 1996).

Liew, Lana, M.D. with Ojeda, Linda, Ph.D. *The Natural Estrogen Diet.* (Alameda, CA: Hunter House, Inc., 1999).

Lopez, D.A., MD, Williams, R.M., M.D., Ph.D., and Miehlke, M., M.D. *Enzymes: The Fountain of Life.* (Charleston, SC: The Neville Press, 1994).

Martin, Raquel. *The Estrogen Alternative.* (Rochester, VT: Healing Arts Press, 1997).

Matsen, Jonn, N.D. *The Mysterious Cause of Illness.* (Canfield, OH: Fischer Publishing, 1987).

McCully, Kilmer, M.D. *The Homocysteine Revolution.* (New Canaan, CT: Keats Publishing, 1997).

McDougall, John A., M.D. *The McDougall Plan.* (Hampton, NJ: New Win Publishing, Inc., 1985).

McDougall, John A., M.D. *The McDougall Program.* (New York, NY: Penguin Books, 1990).

Messina, Mark, Ph.D. and Messina, Virginia, R.D. *The Simple Soybean and Your Health.* (Garden City Park, NY: Avery Publishing, 1994).

Messinger, Lisa. *Why Should I Eat Better?* (New York, NY: Avery Publishers, NY, 1993).

Moran, Victoria. *Get the Fat Out.* (New York, NY: Crown Publishers, 1994).

Morgenthaler, John and Lenard, Lane, Ph.D. *5-HTP: (5 Hydroxytryptophan) The Natural Alternative to Prozac.* (Petaluma, CA: Smart Publications, 1998).

Ojeda, Linda, Ph.D. *Menopause Without Medicine.* (Alameda, CA: Hunter House, Inc. Publishers, 1995).

Ornish, Dean, M.D. *Eat More, Weigh Less.* (New York, NY: Harper Collins, 1997).

Oski, Frank A., M.D. *Don't Drink Your Milk.* (Bruston, NY: Teach Services, Inc. 1983).

Parks, Mary June. *A New You.* (Frankfort, KY: Parks Publishers, 1982).

Parks, Mary June. *Menu and the Mind.* (Frankfort, KY: Parks Publishers, 1986).

Pearl, Bill. *Getting Stronger.* (Shelter Publishing Company, Bolimas, CA.)

Peskin, Brian Scott. *Beyond the Zone.* (Houston, TX: Noble Publishing, 1999).

Quillin, Patrick, Ph.D. *Beating Cancer With Nutrition.* (Tulsa, OK: The Nutrition Times Press, Inc., 1994).

Rockwell, Sally. *Allergy Recipes.* (Seattle, WA: Sally Rockwell Publishing, 1985).

Sahelian, Ray, M.D. *The Stevia Cookbook.* (Garden City Park, NY: Avery Publishing Group, 1999).

Santillo, Humbart, N.D. *Food Enzymes: The Missing Link to Radiant Health.* (Prescott, AZ: Hohm Press, 1987).

Schwartz, Bob. *Diets Still Don't Work!* (Houston, TX: Breakthru Publishing, 1990).

Shelton, Herbert M. *Food Combining Made Easy.* (San Antonio, TX: Willow Publishing, Inc., 1982).

Simontacchi, Carol, C.C.N., M.S. *Your Fat Is Not Your Fault.* (New York, NY: Jeremy P. Tarcher/Putnam 1997).

Strauss, Steven C. and North, Gail. *The Body Signal Secret.* (Emmaus, PA: Rodale Press, 1991).

Steward, H. Leighton, Morrison C. Bethea, M.D., Samuel S. Andrews, M.D., and Luis A. Balart, M.D. *Sugar Busters!* (New York, NY: The Ballantine Publishing Group, 1998).

Tenney, Louise. *Modern Day Plagues.* (Pleasant Grove, UT: Woodland Publishing, Inc. 1994).

Townsley, Cheryl. *Candida Made Simple.* (Littleton, CO: LFH Publishing, 1999).

Townsley, Cheryl. *Cleansing Made Simple.* (Littleton, CO: LFH Publishing, 1997).

Weil, Andrew, M.D. *8 Weeks to Optimum Health.* (New York, NY: Alfred A. Knopf, 1997).

Wright, Jonathan V., M.D. *Dr. Wright's Guide to Healing With Nutrition.* (New Canaan, CT: Keats Publishing, Inc., 1984).

Zimmerman, Marcia, C.N. *The A.D.D. Nutrition Solution: A Drug-Free Thirty-Day Plan.* (New York: NY: Henry Holt and Company, Inc., 1999).

Magazines and Newsletters:

Duncan, Lindsey, C.N., N.D. "Internal Detoxification." *Healthy & Natural Journal,* October 1988.

Duncan, Lindsey, C.N., N.D. Product Information Sheet: Ultimate Weight Loss. NS10165-02. Boulder, Colorado: Nature's Secret, 1998.

Duncan, Lindsey, C.N., N.D. Product Information Sheet: Candistroy. NS10121-02. Boulder, Colorado: Nature's Secret, 1998.

Duncan, Lindsey, C.N., N.D. "Candida Self-Test" *Healthy & Natural Journal,* JS 10073-00.

Nutrition Action Healthletter, Center for Science in the Public Interest, Suite 300, 1875 Connecticut Avenue, N.W., Washington, DC 20009-5728.

Health Alert, Dr. Bruce West, 5 Harris Court, N6, Monterey, CA 93940-5753.

Total Health Magazine, "How To Purify Your Bloodstream," Willa Vae Bowles, February 1987, p. 34.

Total Health Magazine, "Be Good To Your Liver," Willa Vae Bowles, June 1992, pp. 30-32.

Free Government Publications:

"The Surgeon General's Report on Nutrition and Health" by C. Everett Koop, Prima Publishing and Communications, Rocklin, CA 95677, 1988.

"Dietary Goals for the United States: Select Committee on Nutrition and Human Needs," United States Senate, U. S. Government Printing Office, Washington, D.C., February 1977.

"Dietary Guidelines for Americans," U.S. Department of Agriculture, U.S. Department of Health and Human Services, Home and Garden Bulletin No. 232, April, 1986.

"Dietary Guidelines for Americans," U.S. Department of Agriculture, U.S. Department of Health and Human Services, Home and Garden Bulletin No. 232, 1990.

"Dietary Guidelines for Americans," U.S. Department of Agriculture, U.S. Department of Health and Human Services, Fourth Edition, 1995.

"Agriculture Handbook No. 456," Nutritive Value of American Foods in Common Units. U.S. Department of Agriculture, 1975.

"Nutritive Value of Foods," United States Department of Agriculture, Home and Garden Bulletin No. 72, 1981.

"The Food Guide Pyramid, U.S.D.A." Human Nutrition Information Service, August 1992, Leaflet No. 572.

"How To Read The New Food Label," Food and Drug Administration, FDA 93-2260.

"Good Sources of Nutrients," USDA, January 1990.

"Shopping for Food and Making Meals in Minutes." U.S. Department of Agriculture Human Nutrition Information Service. Home and Garden Bulletin No. 232-10.

Data supplied by various food manufacturers and companies. I have made every effort possible to check the accuracy of material quoted and gain permission to copy. If there is any question or a possible mistake in the quoting of any material, necessary changes will be made in future printings.

Recipe Index

Subject Index

F

ORDER FORM

Please Print

Name_____

Address _____

City_____ State _____ Zip _____

Phone _____

E-Mail _____

METHOD OF PAYMENT:

Check _____   **Credit Card** ☐ **Visa OR** ☐ **Mastercard**

Card #_____ Exp. Date _____

Authorization Signature_____

ITEM	QTY.	PRICE
Why Can't I Lose Weight? ($17.95)		
Why Can't I Stay Motivated? ($14.95)		
Why Can't I Lose Weight? COOKBOOK ($17.95)		
SUBTOTAL		
SHIPPING & HANDLING ADD 15%		
TAX		
TOTAL		

Send check or money order to:
  Life Design Nutrition
  Lorrie Medford, C.N.
  P.O. Box 54007
  Tulsa, OK 74155
  918-664-4483
  E-mail orders: lorrie@lifedesignnutrition.com
  www.lifedesignnutrition.com

ORDER FORM

Please Print

Name_____

Address _____

City_____ State _____ Zip _____

Phone _____

E-Mail _____

METHOD OF PAYMENT:

Check _____   Credit Card ☐ Visa OR ☐ Mastercard

Card #_____ Exp. Date _____

Authorization Signature_____

ITEM	QTY.	PRICE
Why Can't I Lose Weight? ($17.95)		
Why Can't I Stay Motivated? ($14.95)		
Why Can't I Lose Weight? COOKBOOK ($17.95)		
SUBTOTAL		
SHIPPING & HANDLING ADD 15%		
TAX		
TOTAL		

Send check or money order to:
    Life Design Nutrition
    Lorrie Medford, C.N.
    P.O. Box 54007
    Tulsa, OK 74155
    918-664-4483
    E-mail orders: lorrie@lifedesignnutrition.com
    www.lifedesignnutrition.com

ORDER FORM

Please Print

Name_____

Address _____

City_____ State _____ Zip _____

Phone _____

E-Mail _____

METHOD OF PAYMENT:

Check _____   **Credit Card** ☐ **Visa OR** ☐ **Mastercard**

Card #_____ Exp. Date _____

Authorization Signature_____

ITEM	QTY.	PRICE
Why Can't I Lose Weight? ($17.95)		
Why Can't I Stay Motivated? ($14.95)		
Why Can't I Lose Weight? COOKBOOK ($17.95)		
SUBTOTAL		
SHIPPING & HANDLING ADD 15%		
TAX		
TOTAL		

Send check or money order to:
  Life Design Nutrition
  Lorrie Medford, C.N.
  P.O. Box 54007
  Tulsa, OK 74155
  918-664-4483
  E-mail orders: lorrie@lifedesignnutrition.com
  www.lifedesignnutrition.com